YOU ARE WHOLE

The Breast Cancer Confidence Project

Portraits and Stories of Breast Cancer Survivors and Thrivers

Photography by Jolana Hollister
Book Design by Gibrana Nemer
Edited by Michaela Raes

BREAST CANCER Confidence PROJECT

First Edition

Published by The Breast Cancer Confidence Project
Rochester, New York
www.BreastCancerConfidence.com

ISBN (Hardcover): 978-1-7338561-1-9

Disclaimer: The stories and experiences shared in this book are personal to each contributor. This book is intended for inspiration and support only. It is not a substitute for professional medical advice, diagnosis, or treatment. Always seek the guidance of your physician or other qualified health provider with any questions regarding your health.

Photography by Jolana Hollister
Book design by Gibrana Nemer
Cover art by Gibrana Nemer
Edited by Michaela Raes

Profits from this book directly support the mission of the Breast Cancer Confidence Project.

Printed in the United States of America

Table of Contents

PREFACE

There is a moment—**sometimes fleeting, sometimes drawn out—when a woman looks in the mirror and struggles to see beauty in her reflection; struggles to see past what she believes to be her imperfections.**

This is a reality for women across all ages, races, and backgrounds. Now imagine that same woman hearing words no one ever wants to hear: You have Breast Cancer. That same woman facing breast cancer looks in the mirror and no longer recognizes herself.

The reflection staring back may bear scars, changed contours, or a body altered by surgery, treatment, and survival. But behind that reflection is something cancer can never take away: wholeness.

You Are Whole was born from this truth. It is a collection of stories and portraits of 26 remarkable women—each from different backgrounds, with different journeys, but united by the strength to reclaim their bodies, their beauty, and their confidence.

Through the intimate lens of boudoir photography, these pages capture not just images, but resilience, defiance, and self-love in its most profound form.

Sharing these portraits with the world is an act of bravery. The women in this book have chosen vulnerability not just for themselves, but for every woman who has ever questioned her own worth because of the changes her body has endured. By baring their scars, they are breaking down antiquated societal beauty standards, normalizing difference, and proving that true beauty is not about perfection— it lies in the imperfect, in what makes us different, and in our authenticity to ourselves. Their courage paves the way for future generations to embrace their bodies without shame and to see transformation not as loss, but as a testament to survival and resilience.

This book is an extension of the mission behind the Breast Cancer Confidence Project, a nonprofit dedicated to healing the body image and self-esteem of breast cancer survivors. Its work focuses on restoring confidence through transformative portrait experiences, showing women that they are not broken, not incomplete—but powerful, radiant, and whole.

We believe that beauty is not defined by society's expectations, but by the courage it takes to embrace oneself fully- scars and all.

To every woman who has ever felt lost in her own skin—whether from breast cancer or any other life event that changed the way you see yourself—this book is for you. May these portraits and stories remind you that you are not alone. May they offer hope when you need it most. And may they help you see yourself through the eyes of love, strength, and undeniable beauty.

Remember: You are whole. You always have been.

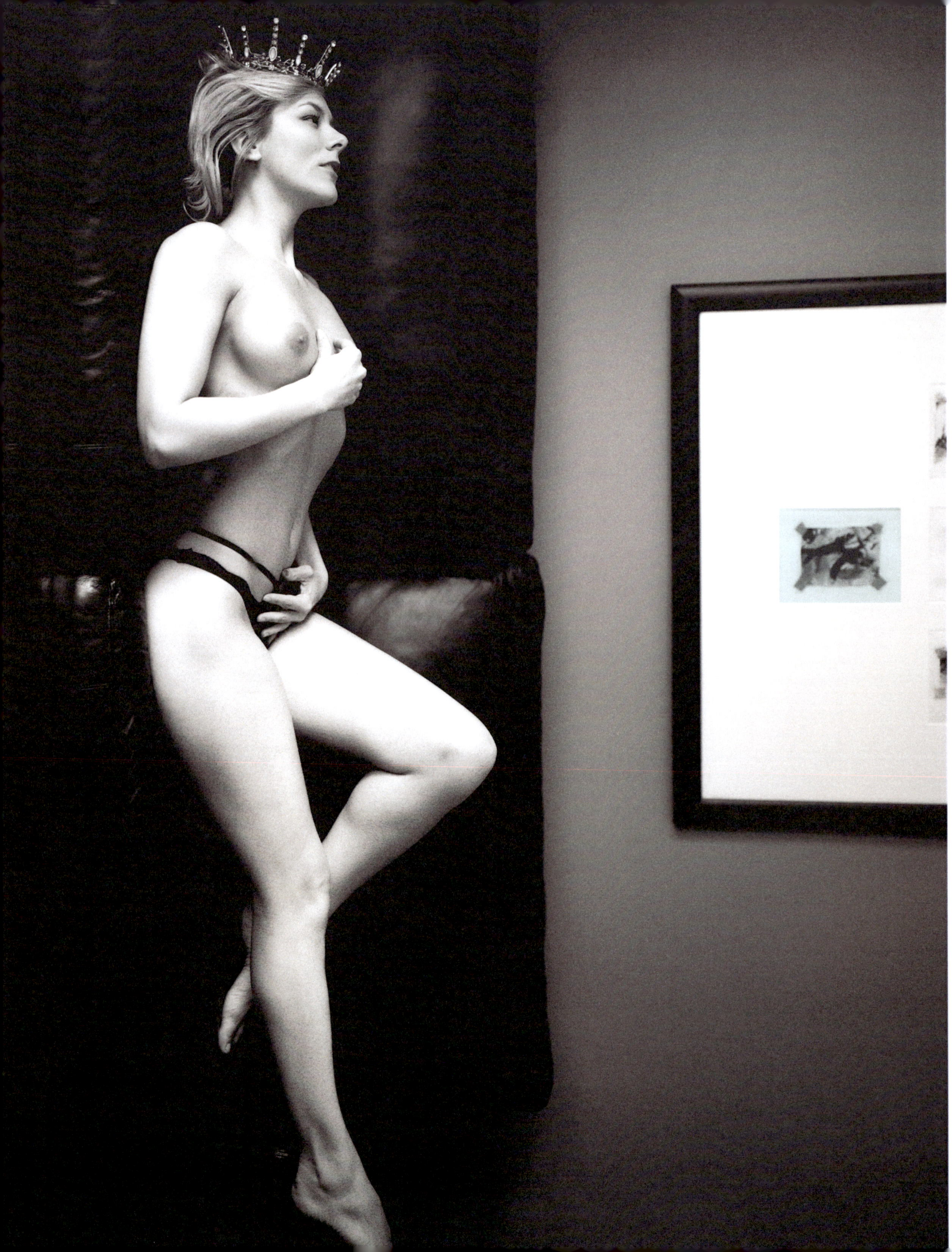

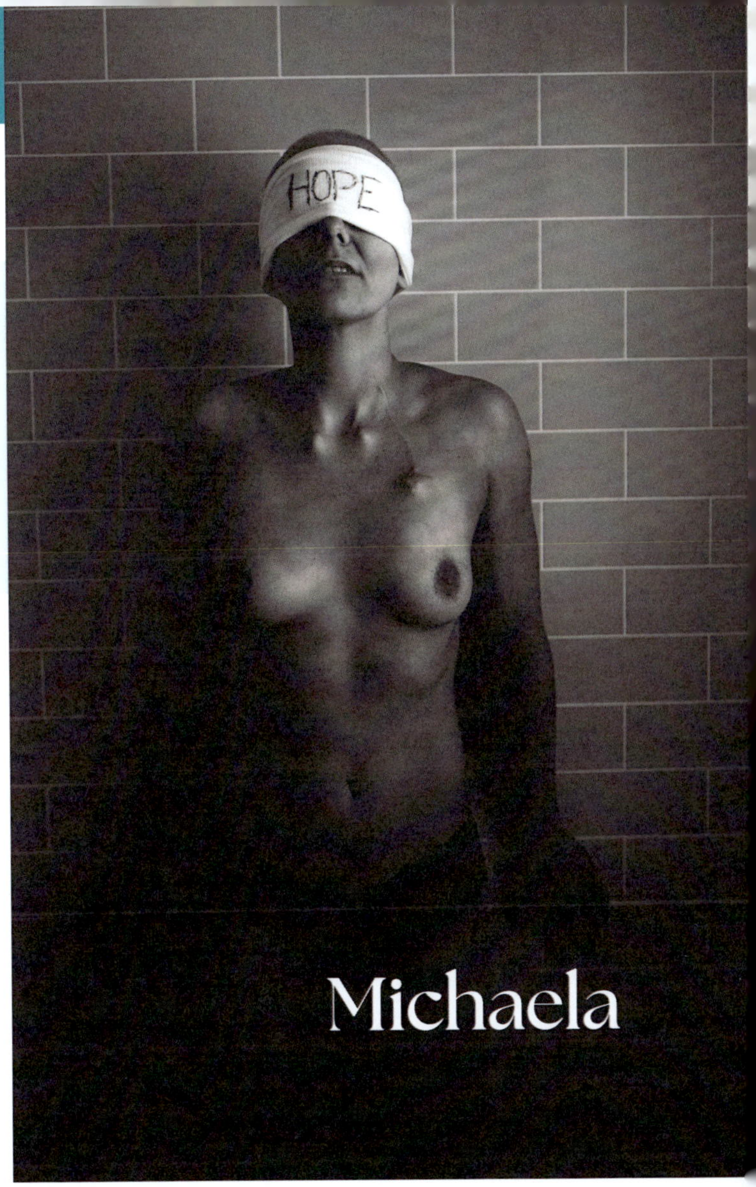

Michaela

Diagnosis: *Stage IIB Triple Negative, Metaplastic Breast Cancer.*
Age Diagnosed: *28*
Treatments Received: *Lumpectomy, Chemotherapy, Double Mastectomy, Implant Reconstruction.*
Age at time of photographs: *28-30*
Stage at time of photographs: *Before, during, and after.*
Region: *Central New York.*
Social Media: *@michaela.camille1*

I was in my late 20s when...

I heard the words no woman ever wants to hear: "You have breast cancer."

In the days after diagnosis, fear consumed me—not just of the disease, but of what it would do to my body.

I braced myself for the day that I'd see a stranger in the mirror.

Desperate to preserve a version of myself I feared would soon be lost, I scheduled a boudoir photoshoot just days before surgery.

As treatment unfolded, something unexpected happened.

Even as chemotherapy drained me and surgeries reshaped me, I still recognized my reflection, and my body refused to surrender. Instead of feeling broken, I felt resilient.

I saw strength where I thought I would see loss, and I was overwhelmed with gratitude for the body that carried me through my darkest days.

That realization sparked a mission to offer the reassurance that I had once needed, and to show women facing breast cancer the power of changing perceptions.

Breast Cancer Confidence Project was created to empower survivors to embrace their bodies, remind them that beauty comes in many forms, and prove that confidence does not need to be lost with a diagnosis.

It's been five years since my diagnosis, and I am still grateful for my body, for my transformation, and for this chance to help others reclaim their confidence after cancer.

If you are facing this diagnosis, know this:

You are strong.

You are whole.

And you are beautiful,

exactly as you are.

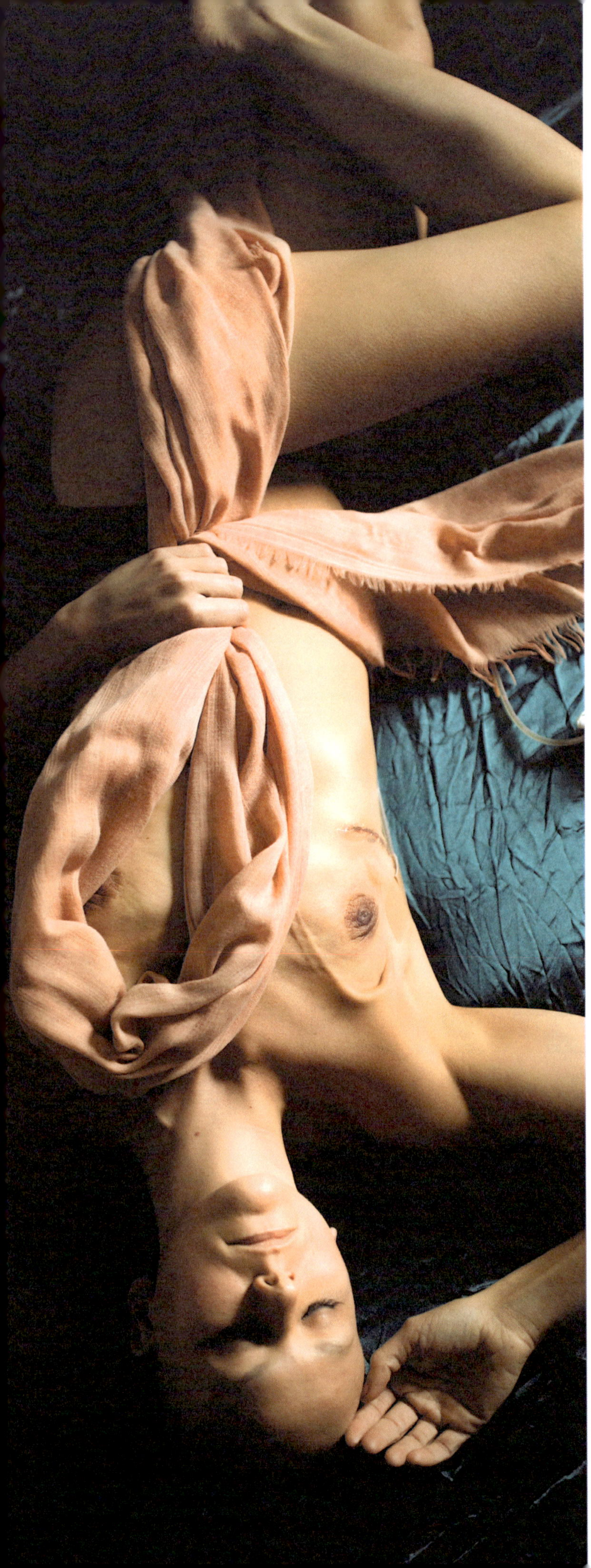
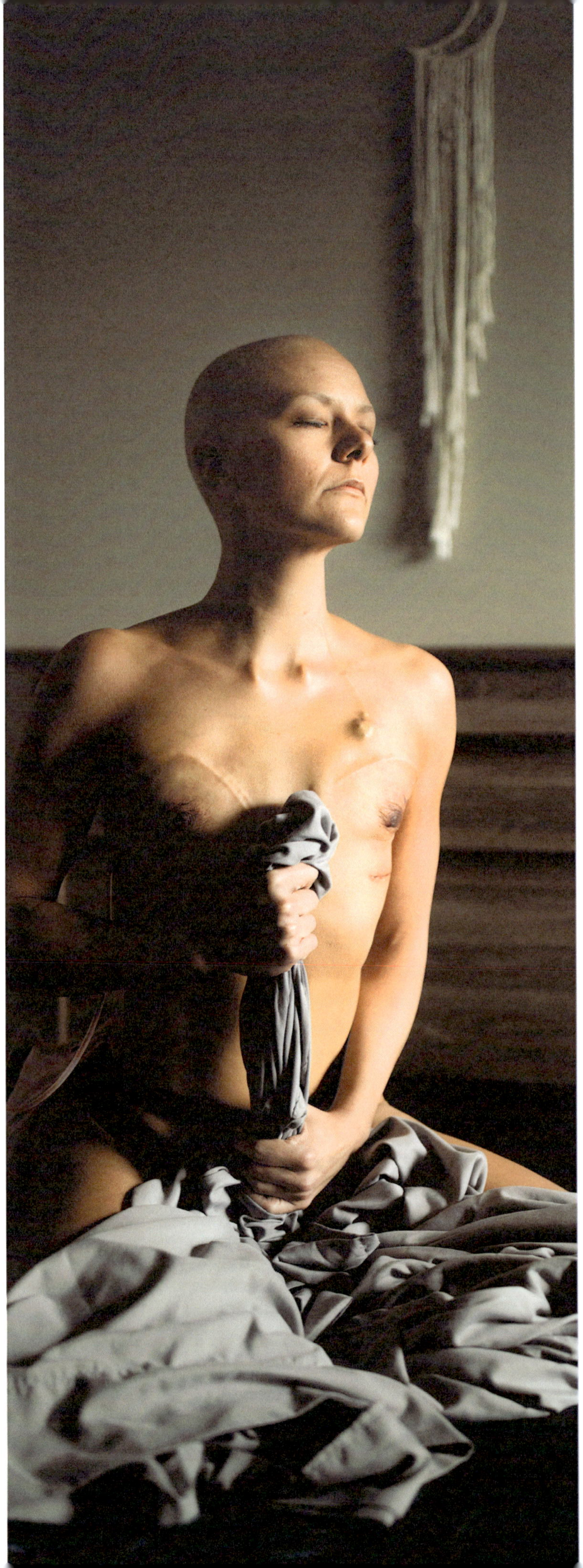

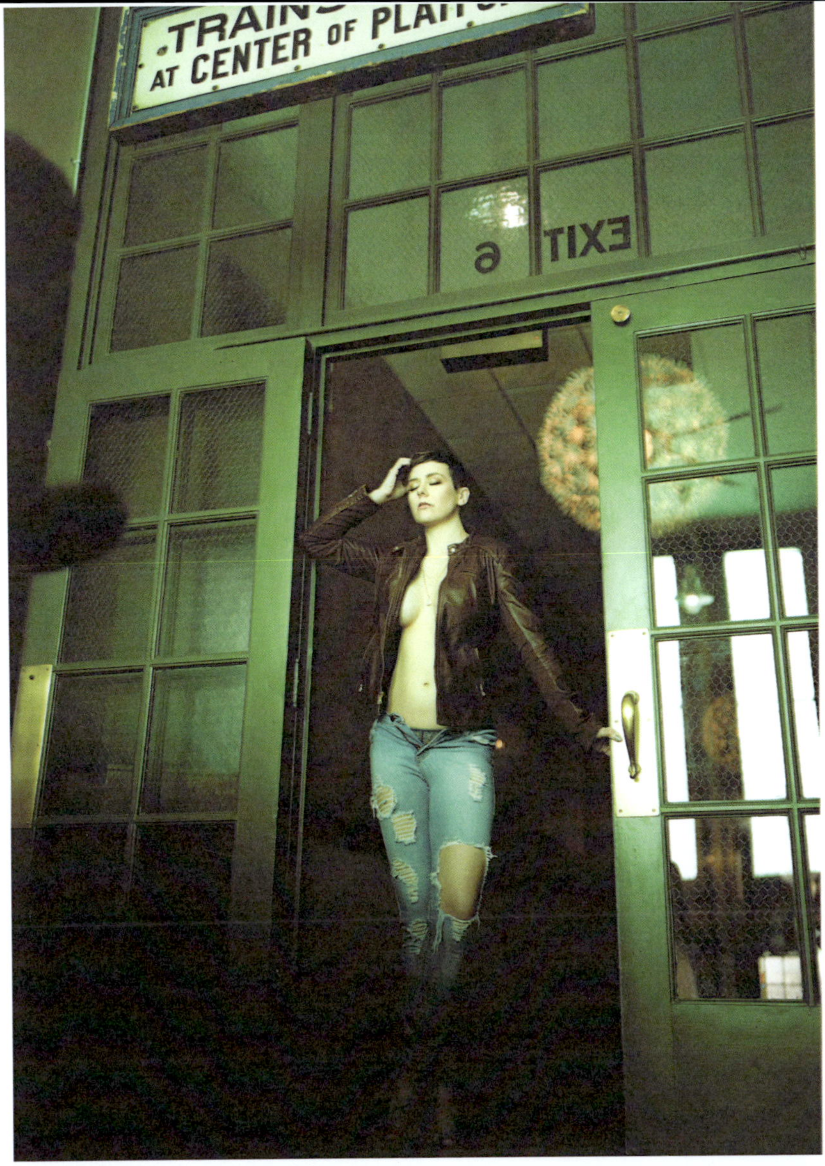
AT CENTER OF
EXIT 6

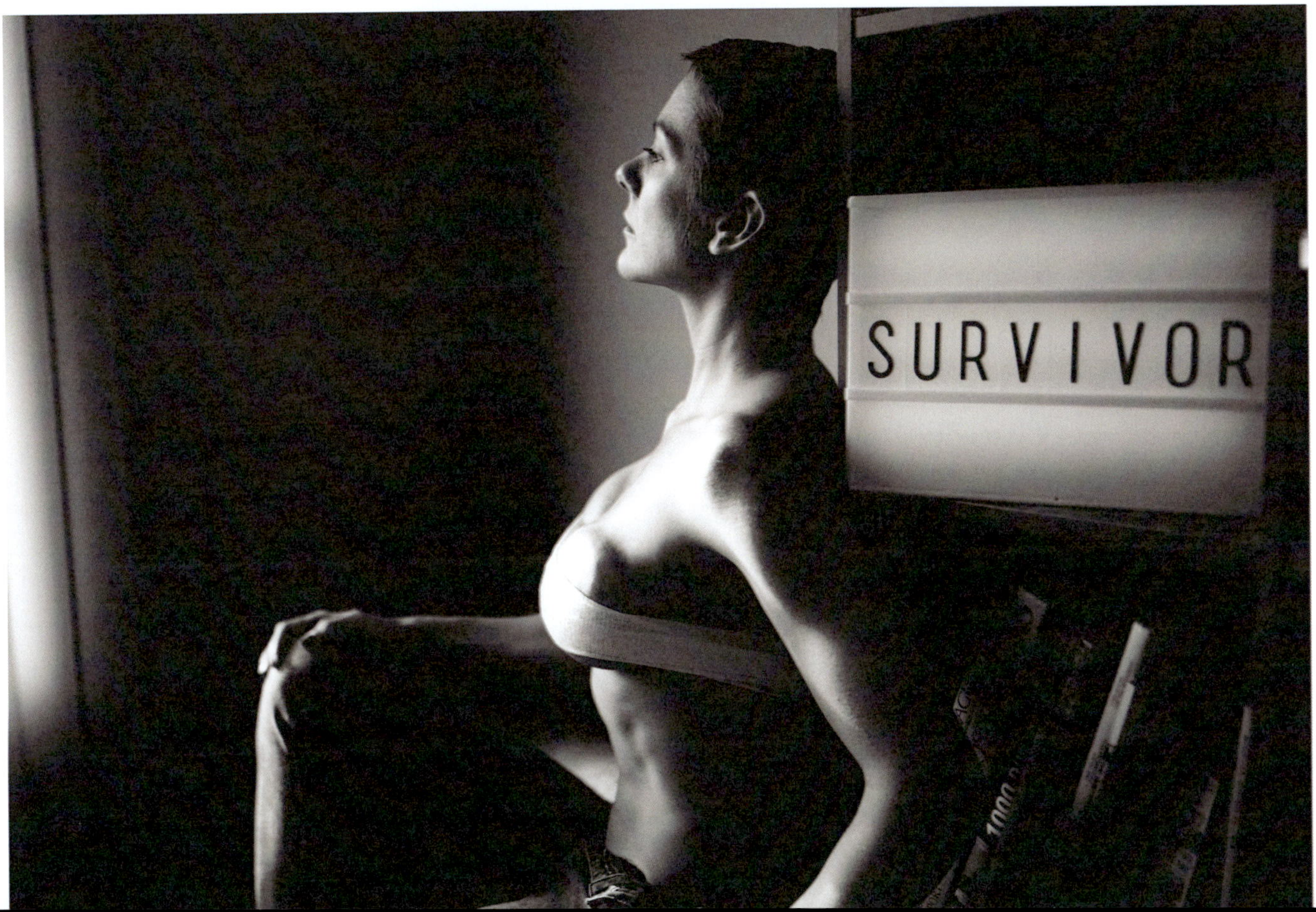
SURVIVOR

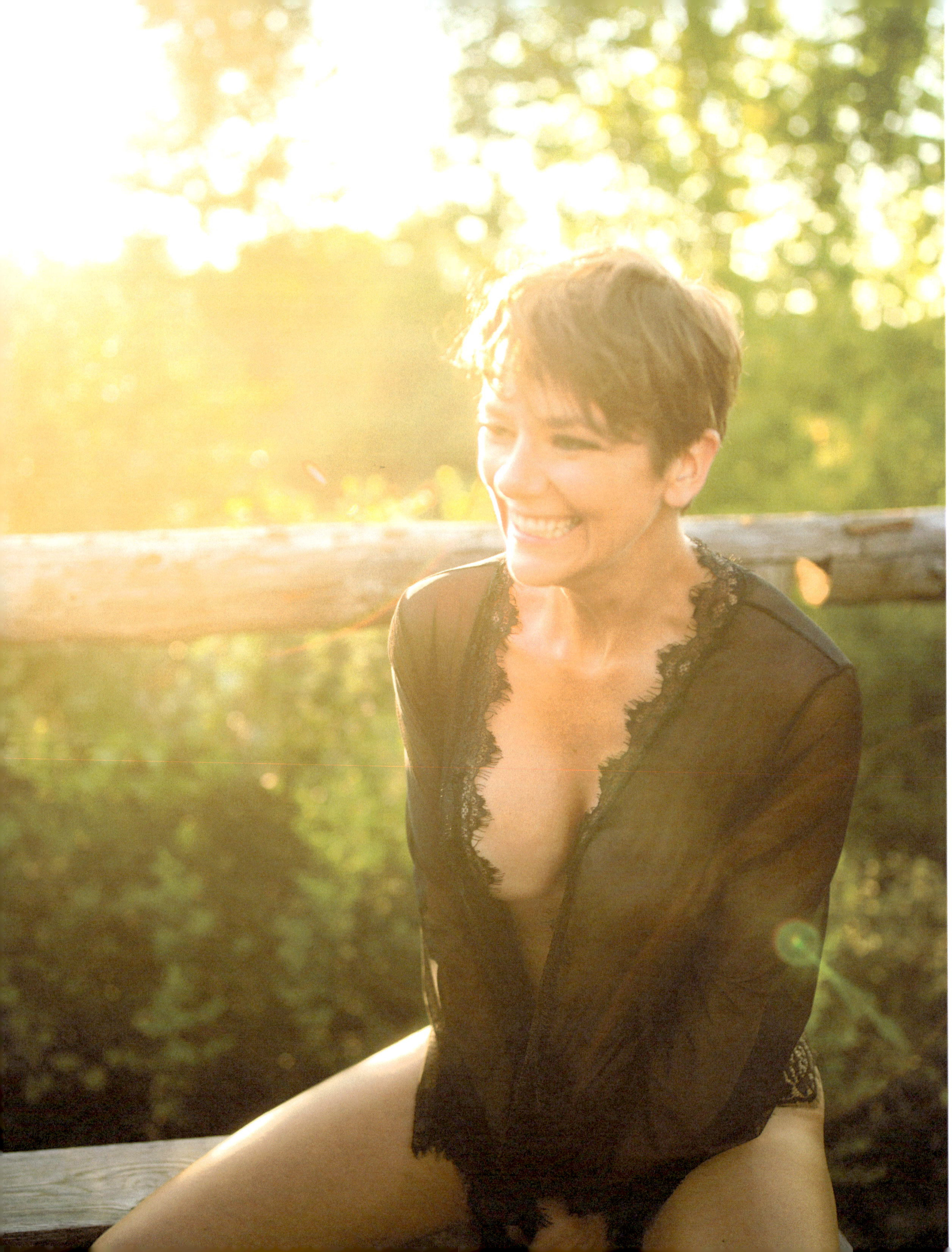

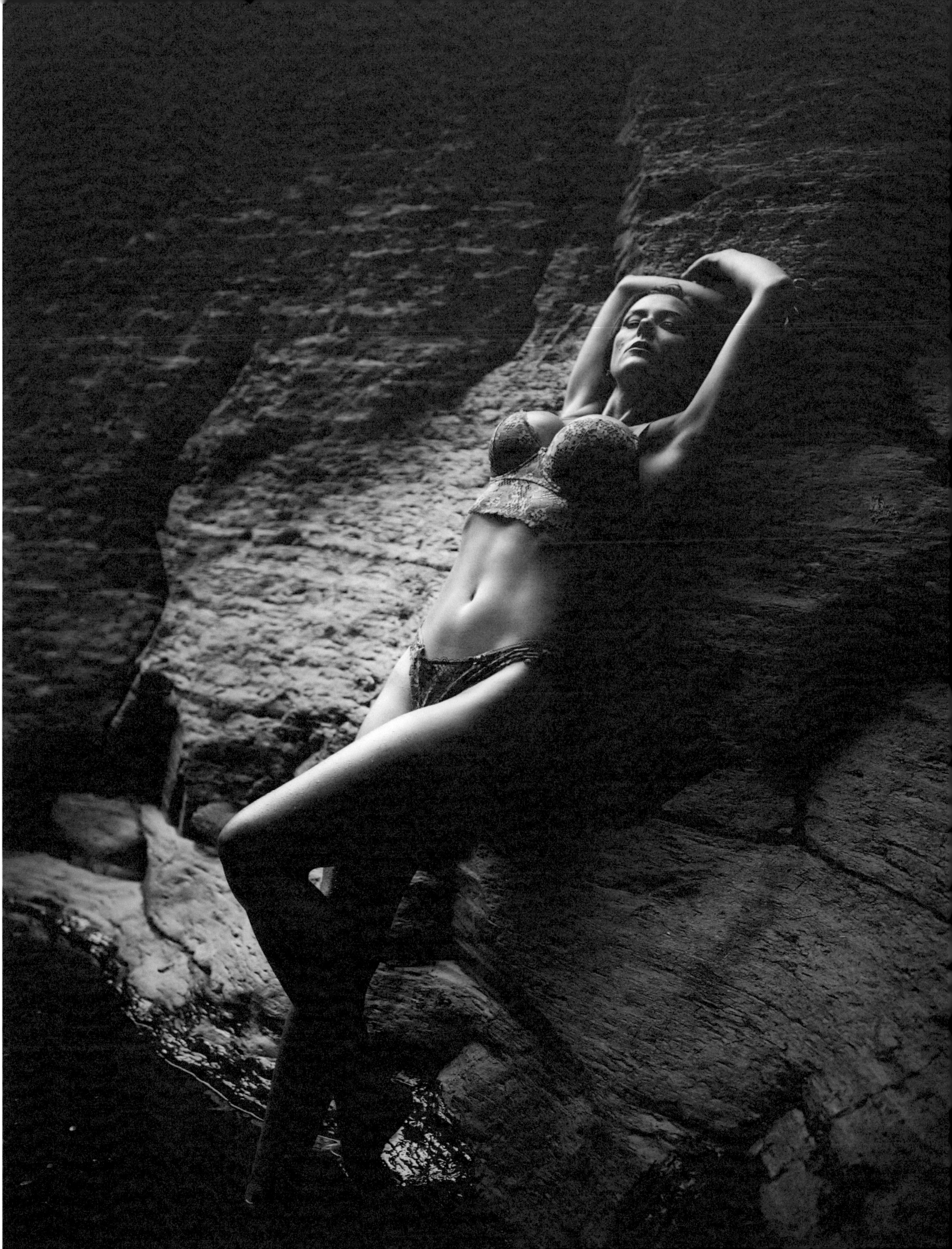

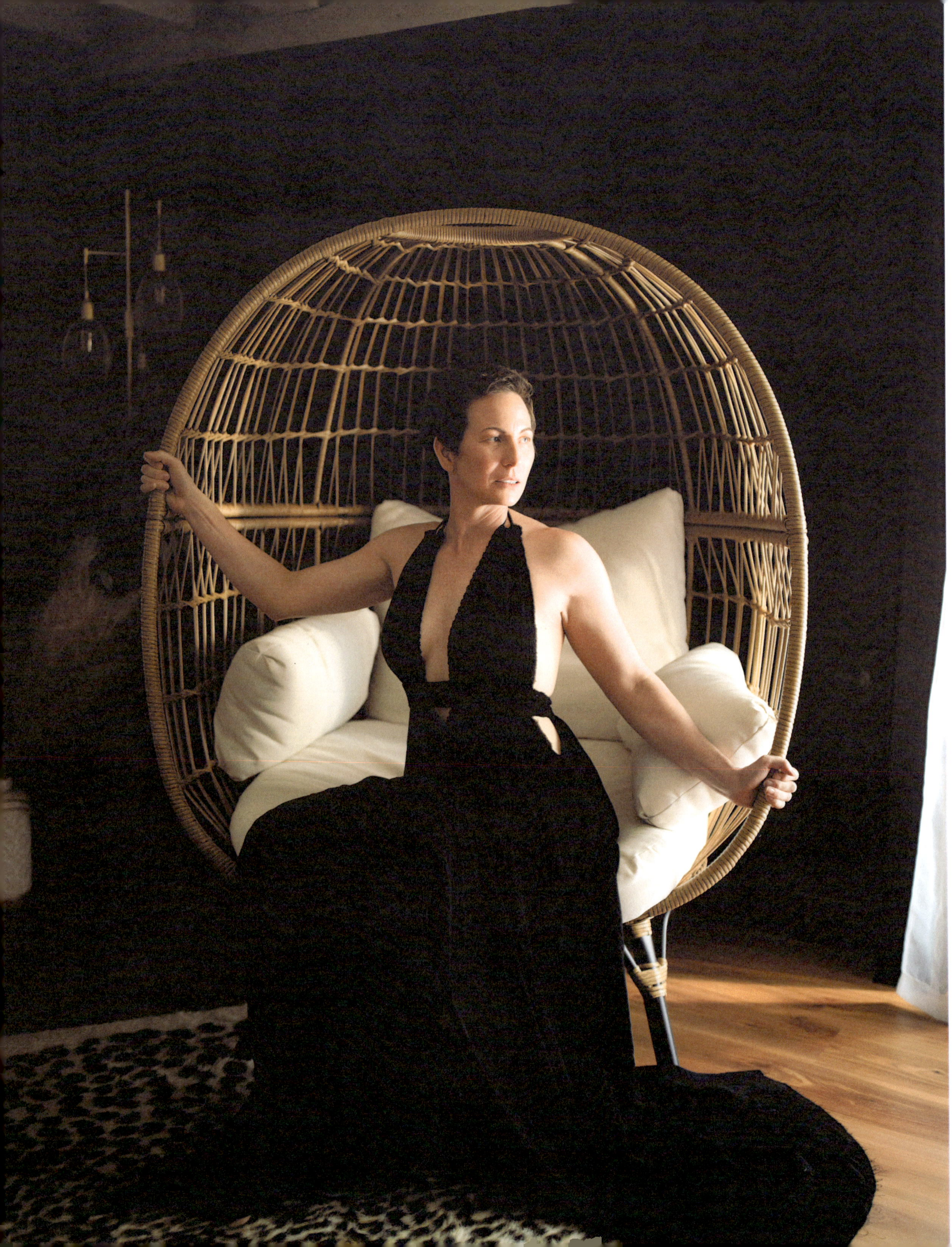

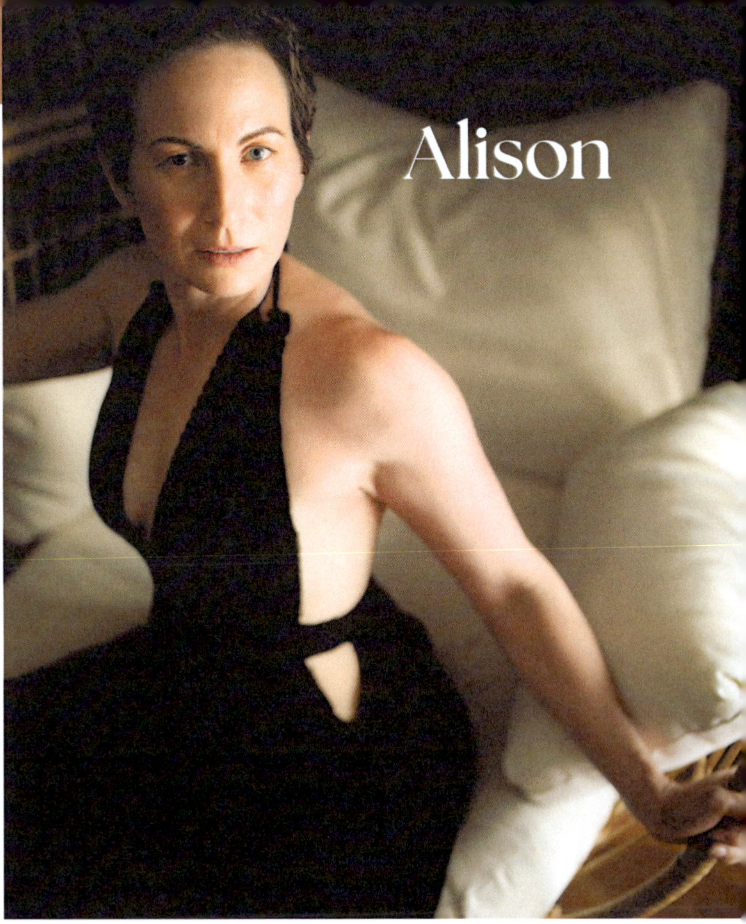

Diagnosis: *Stage 1a hormone positive breast cancer*
Age Diagnosed: *40*
Treatments Received: *Chemo, mastectomy, oopherectomy and total hysterectomy, hormone blocker*
Age at time of photographs: *41*
Stage at time of photographs: *NED*
Region: *Pacific Northwest*

One evening I noticed a change in the mirror.

I wasn't too worried -- I was an athlete and had hoped to complete a triathlon in the near future, had no family history, no real risk factors (that I knew of). I mean, I bought all the organic things so I could avoid getting cancer. Cancer wasn't on my radar.

I was told I had hormone-positive breast cancer. So much has changed in my life since that moment.

The many firsts: MRI, surgery/anesthesia (x2), JP drains (x2), post-op complications (x2), chemotherapy (x4), a bald head, menopause, perimenopause, medications, etc. etc.

And, all the gratitude.
Gratitude.

Chemo humbled, and increased my tolerance for discomfort, taught self-grace, resilience, GRIT.
Baldness gifted me perspective, and strength, and some great earrings.

Support, especially from my husband and my female tribe, deeply inspires me to a) accept the help and b) pay it forward.

Fear reminds me to breath, to live every day with presence; to go to the beach, get my hands in the dirt and feet dirty in sand, have tea with friends, hug
my sweet daughter and husband, my rocks.

The incredible women I've met so far on this journey, fellow breast cancer survivors and thrivers, inspire me to LIVE. With purpose. In awe. To DANCE, rediscover and learn new creative expressions, take care of my body/mind/soul, laugh, love on my fur babies, travel, go to the concert, get the tattoo, say "yes" to adventure, speak my mind, to not sweat the small stuff. I could go on and on.

Just, some things I now know from a different lens: Monthly checks - don't forget them ("feel it on the first"). Yes, men too. Get to know your body.

Get preventative care. Speak up if you notice ANYTHING different. Demand further workup, scans. Ask the questions. Get the 2nd and 3rd opinions, whatever it takes to become informed. Healthcare is extremely challenging/stressful to navigate (and I'm privileged).

Know your family health history.

Don't assume a woman had breast surgery because she wanted to. And, be aware of the fact that reconstruction is an entirely different thing than augmentation. And, some women decide to forgo reconstruction and go "flat". For most, treatment continues for years and can cause side effects that impact quality of life.

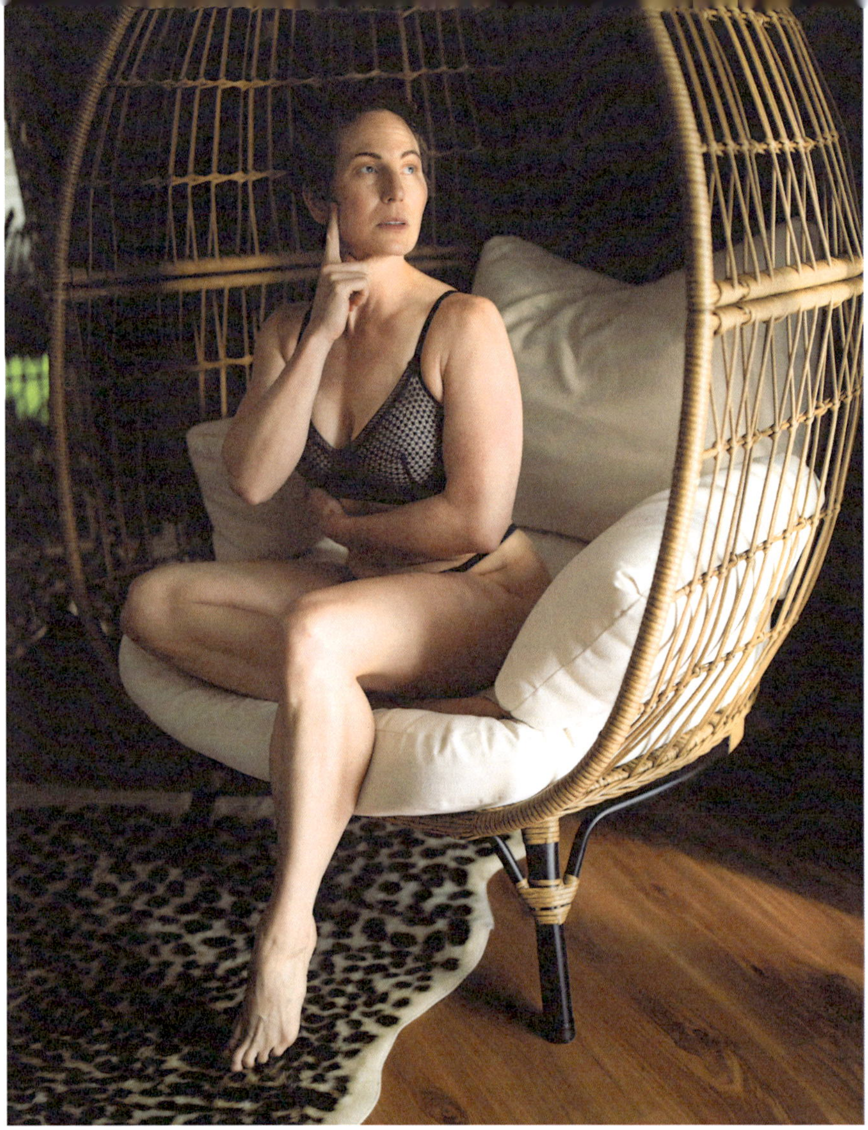

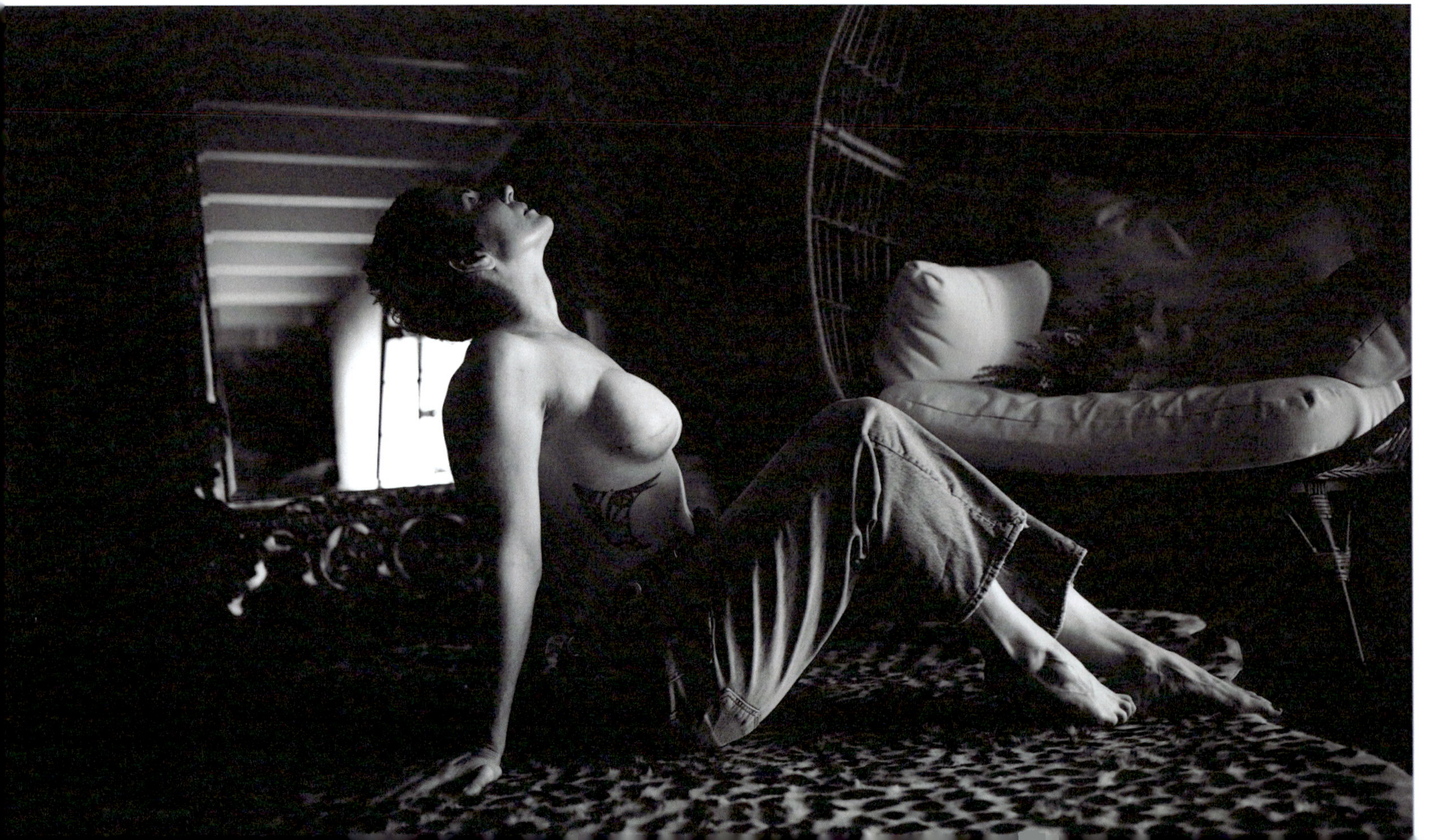

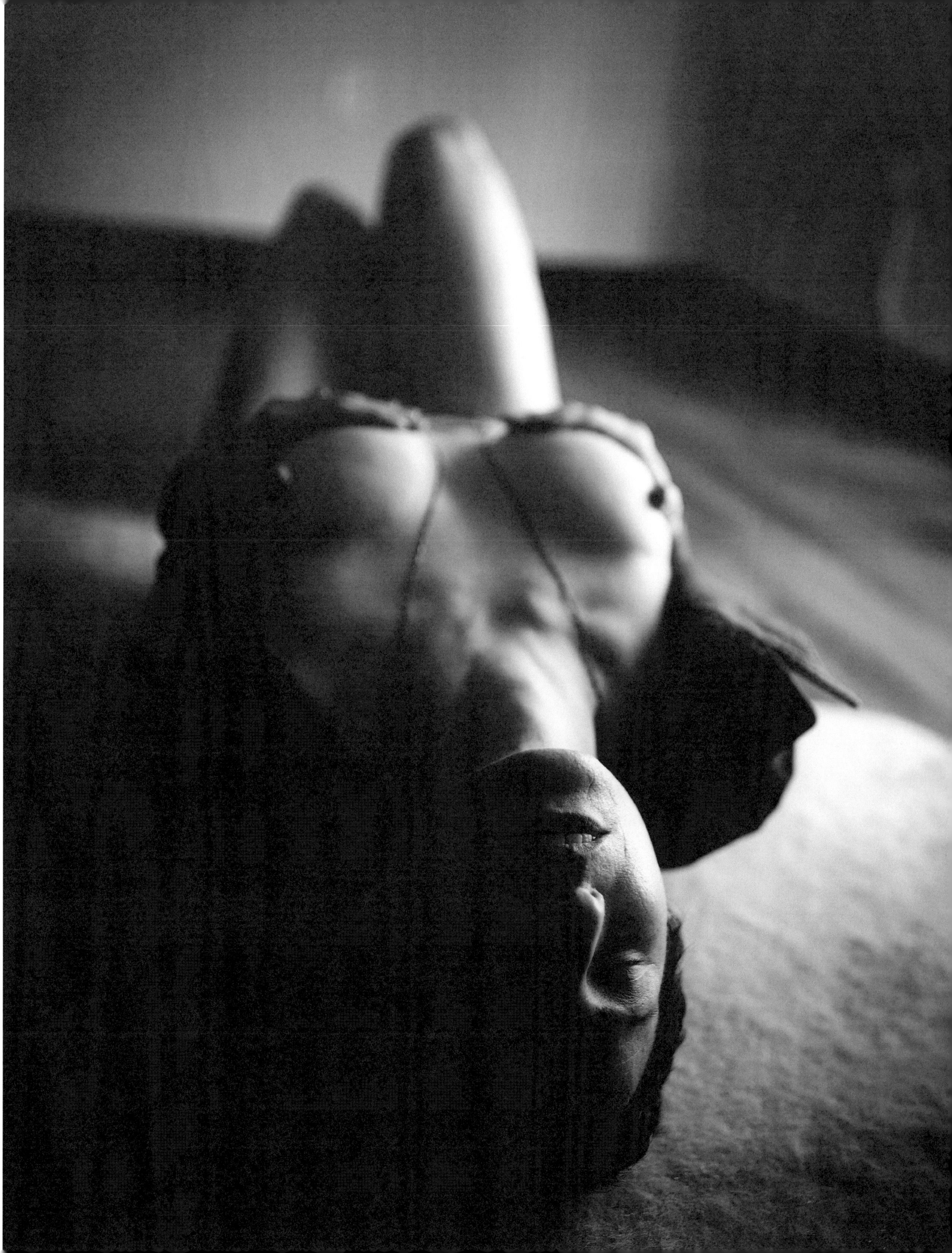

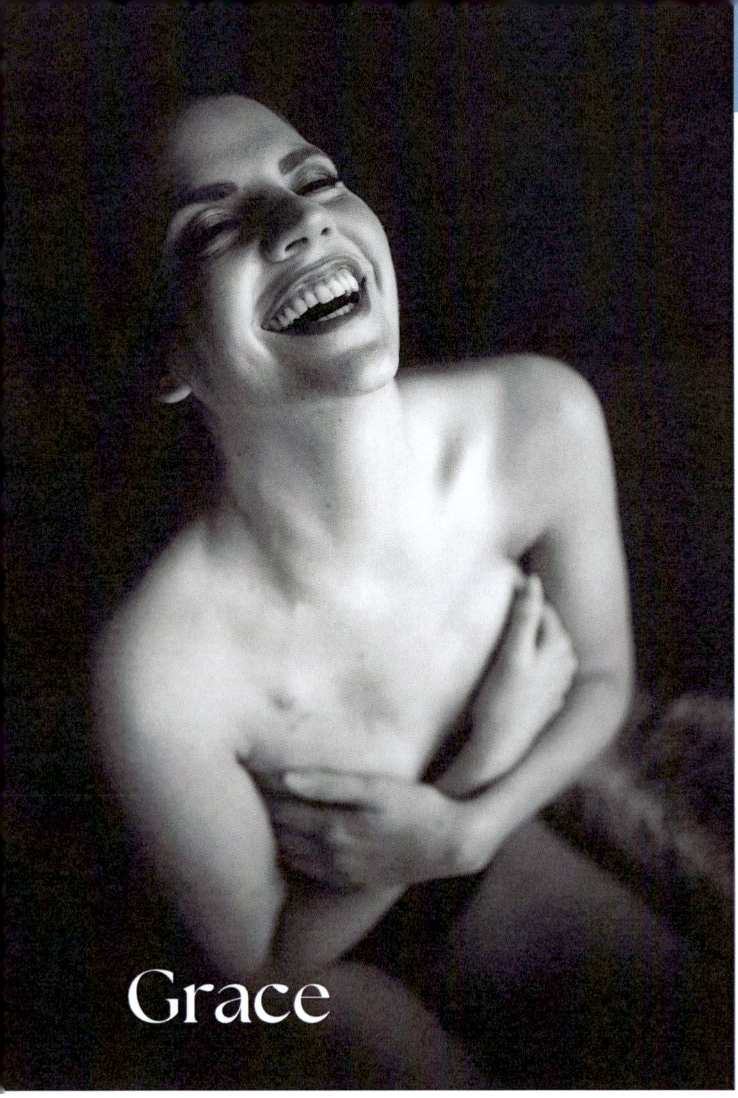

Grace

Diagnosis: *Stage 2 Triple Negative Breast Cancer.*
Age Diagnosed: *30*
Treatments Received: *Keynote 522 Regimen - Chemotherapy, Immunotherapy and Double Mastectomy.*
Age at time of photographs: *31*
Stage at time of photographs: *One month post double mastectomy with tissue expanders.*
Region: *Chicago, IL*

Whenever I look at my body and catch myself critiquing it, I remind myself "This body fought and beat cancer."

That simple sentence has become a powerful tool to help me reframe those negative thoughts and honor my body that endured so much to keep me alive.

There's something especially cruel and ironic about how breast cancer targets the parts of our body that are equated with femininity: our breasts and our hair. Losing these didn't make me less of a woman. If anything, it showed the strength and resiliency that was there all along.

At the beginning of my diagnosis, I started practicing gratitude more regularly. At first it felt unnatural and even a little silly. I was questioning, what could I possibly feel grateful for as I was just diagnosed with breast cancer at 30?!

I felt like I was repeating the same things over and over. But slowly as I continued to practice, I noticed it coming more naturally.

When times were especially tough or there was a setback with treatment, I was able to shift my mindset more easily and quickly register what I was grateful for in that moment. Gratitude didn't erase the pain, but it gave me a way through it. Practicing gratitude truly is a practice! It's like a muscle, the more you use it, the stronger it gets.

When I was preparing for my double mastectomy, there were so many choices to make, it was overwhelming. This was finally something that I felt I had control over when so much of my life felt out of control.

I met with multiple surgeons, weighed my options: Over or under the muscle? Keep my nipples or remove them? What size implants? It felt like a lot of pressure to make the "right" decision. With good intentions, people would often say "At least you'll get great new boobs out of this!" All I wanted was to keep my old boobs.

A double mastectomy with reconstruction is not the same as breast augmentation. They are completely different surgeries and outcomes. I wish I had a better understanding of that going into my double mastectomy.

What I quickly realized is the new boobs will have flaws just like the "originals" had. The asymmetry and stretch marks would be traded for some rippling, scars, and lack of sensation.

It will take time to accept these changes, just like it took time to accept the body I had before cancer.

It's still a work in progress to love and accept these new girls, but these imperfections show my strength and tell the story of what I went through.

Diagnosis: *Triple Postiive Breast Cancer.*
Age Diagnosed: *28*
Treatments Received: *6 rounds TCHP Chemo, double mastectomy, 30 rounds radiation.*
Age at time of photographs: *29*
Stage at time of photographs: *Stage II*
Region: *Midwest*

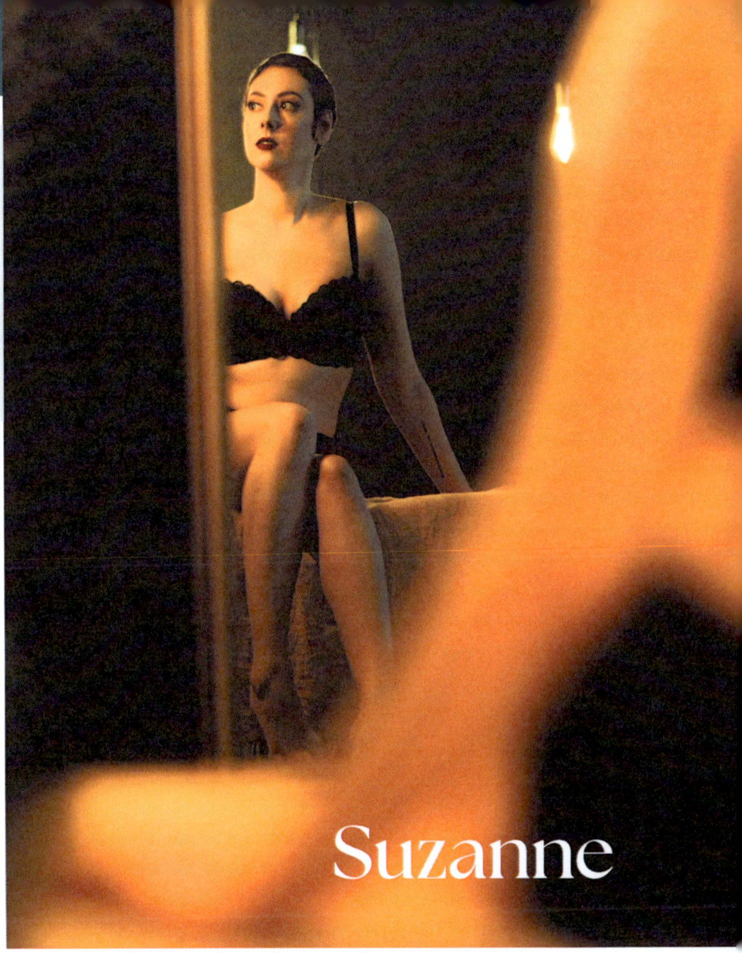

Even before cancer, I had trouble loving my body.

I grew up surrounded by purity culture, which taught me that my body was sinful and tempting, and needed to be covered up in order to "protect" others. It was a long journey for me to come to a place where I felt comfortable allowing my body to just be, to just exist in the world, without all of that baggage attached to it.

Losing your sense of self as you become just another patient, just another body, just another cancerous entity is a real problem, but in a way, the cavalierness with which everyone else treated my boobs allowed me to let go of some of my shame.

Growing up, breasts were seen as the end all, be all of female sexuality.

They were shrouded in a certain scandalous mystique, imbued with the power to wreck marriages, households, and piety.

Cancer taught me that that's not true! Boobs are just boobs. To my doctors, they were simply another part of the human body, as regular and mundane as a leg or arm.

That's not to say that losing my breasts and my old body wasn't a struggle; it very much was.

I miss my old physique, the one without the scars, the implants, the port, and the numbness.

I miss the limberness and flexibility I had before surgery, radiation, and hormone therapy took it away.

But hidden in all of this mess is a deeper message, that bodies and boobs and beauty are not all that we are. I am much more than my cancer; I am much more than my body! I am a complex individual filled with goals, dreams, love, laughter, frustration, anger, fear, passion, and life.

I am reminded of Walt Whitman's Song of Myself: "I am large, I contain multitudes." We all contain multitudes.

I wouldn't say I love my body now. It did, after all, try to kill me.

But I appreciate it as a vessel that allows me to continue experiencing life, which I love more than anything. I've come to look at my body in a more objective way, and I think that's good for me. Instead of my body being an end in itself, I treat it more as a means to an end–or a beginning.

My scars, implants, and port allow me to keep traveling, creating, and existing. My body lets me live. My body lets me love. I am thankful for that, and that is enough.

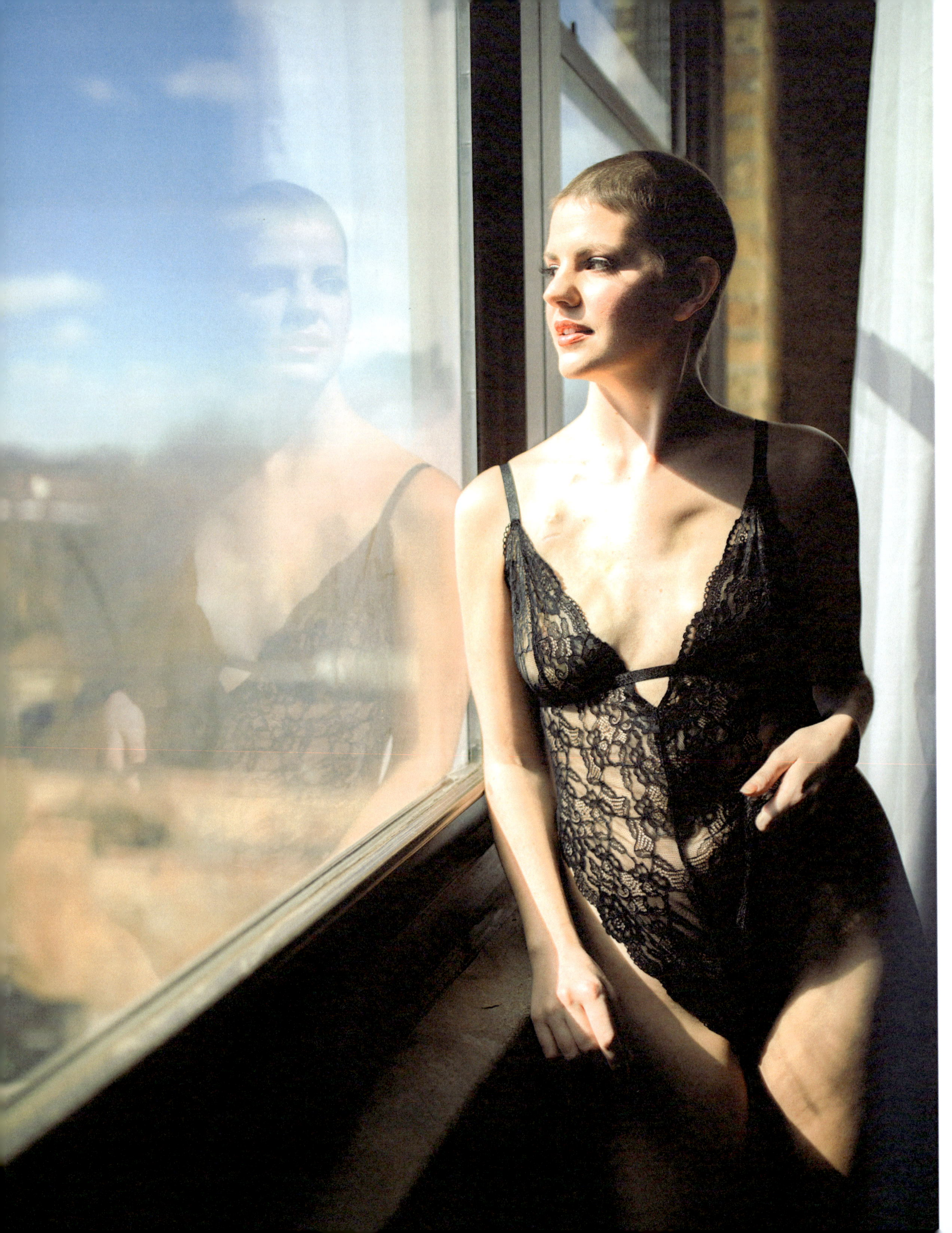

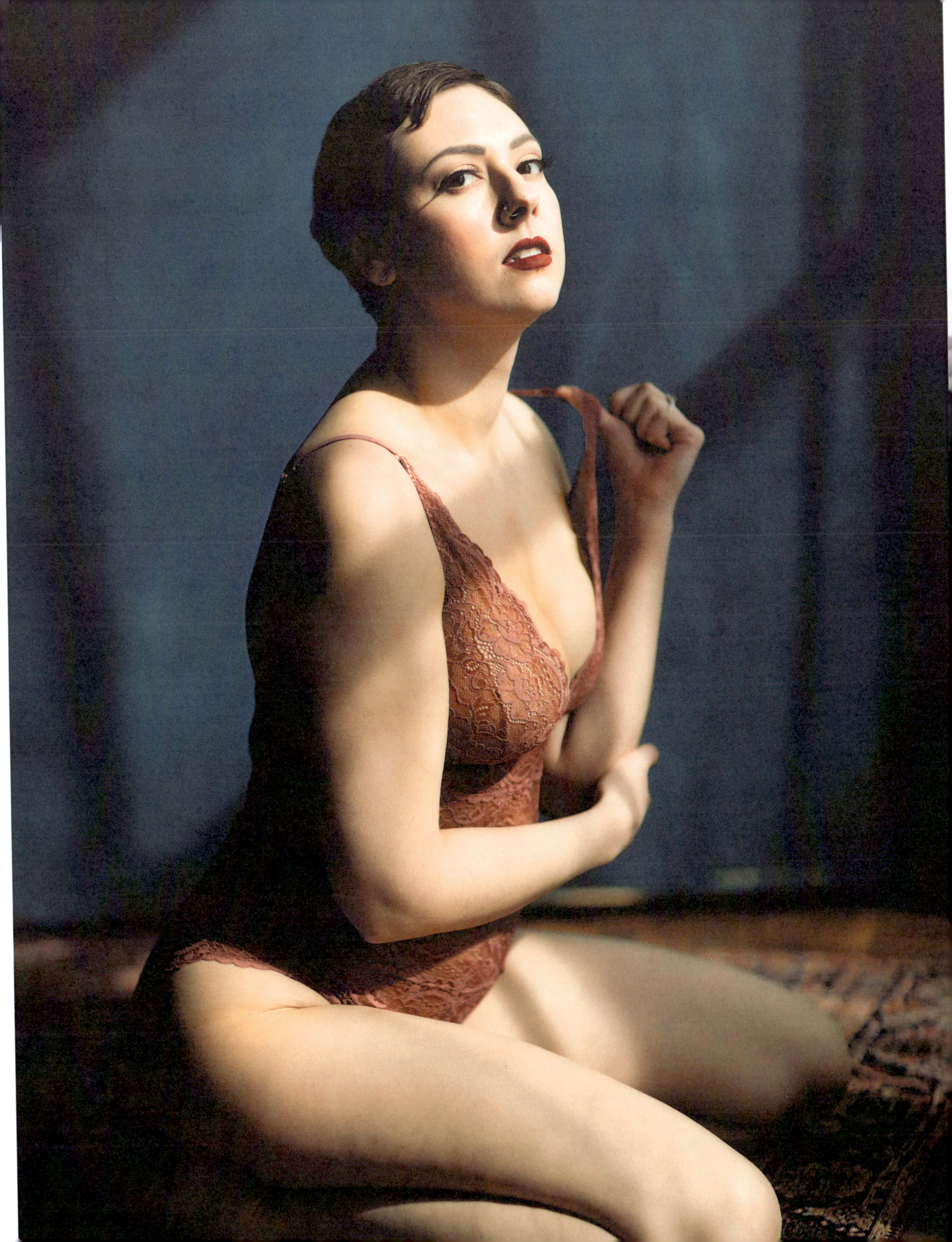

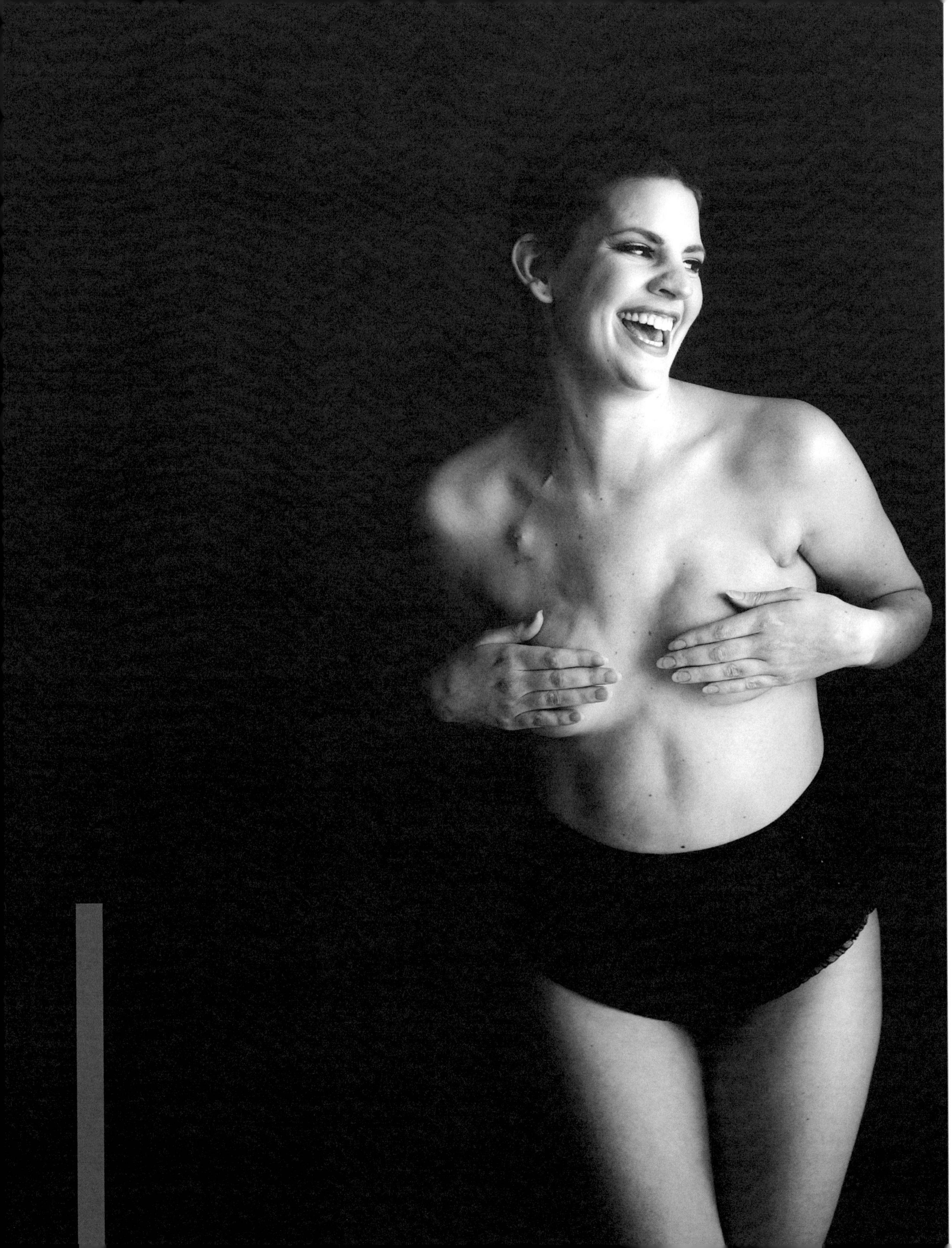

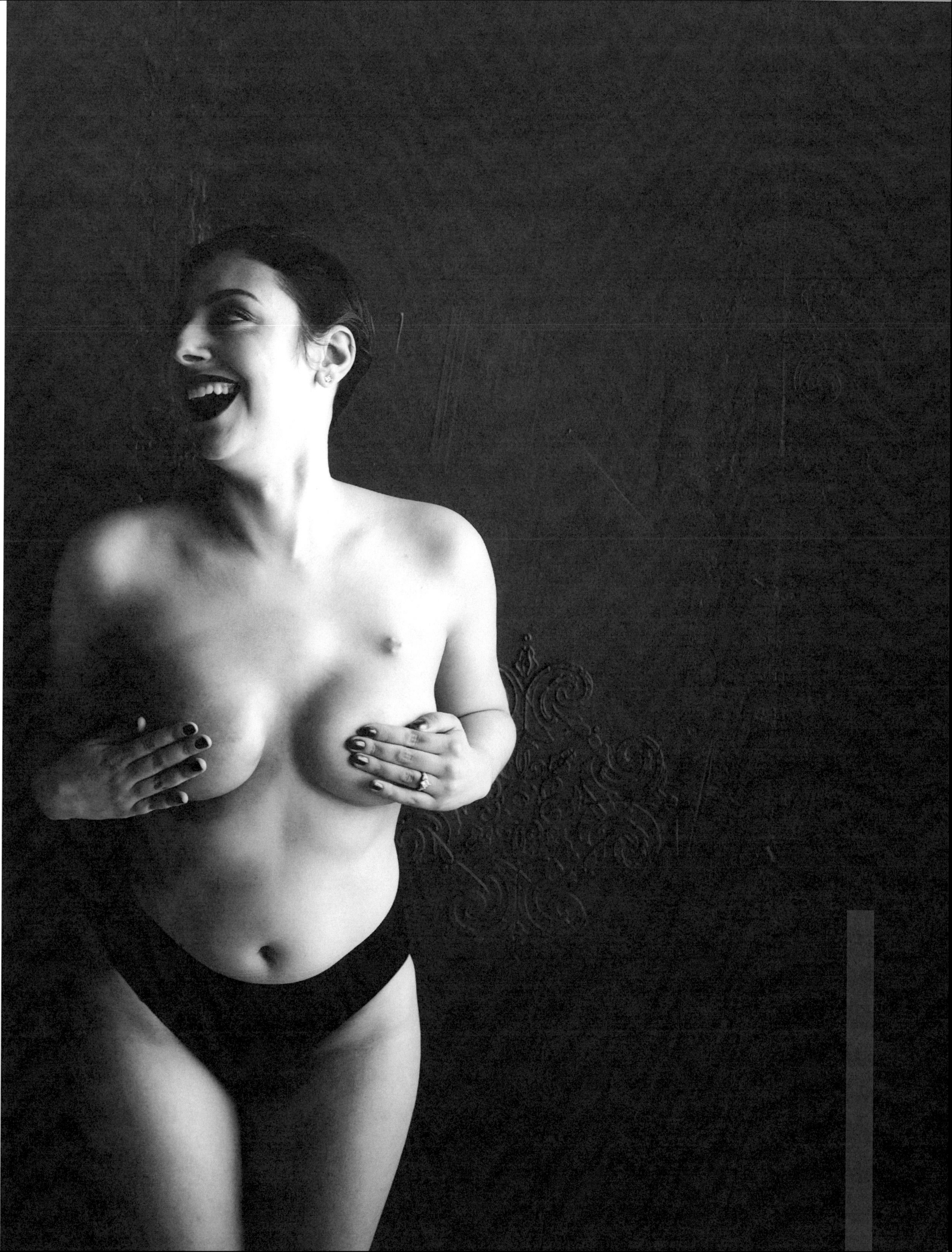

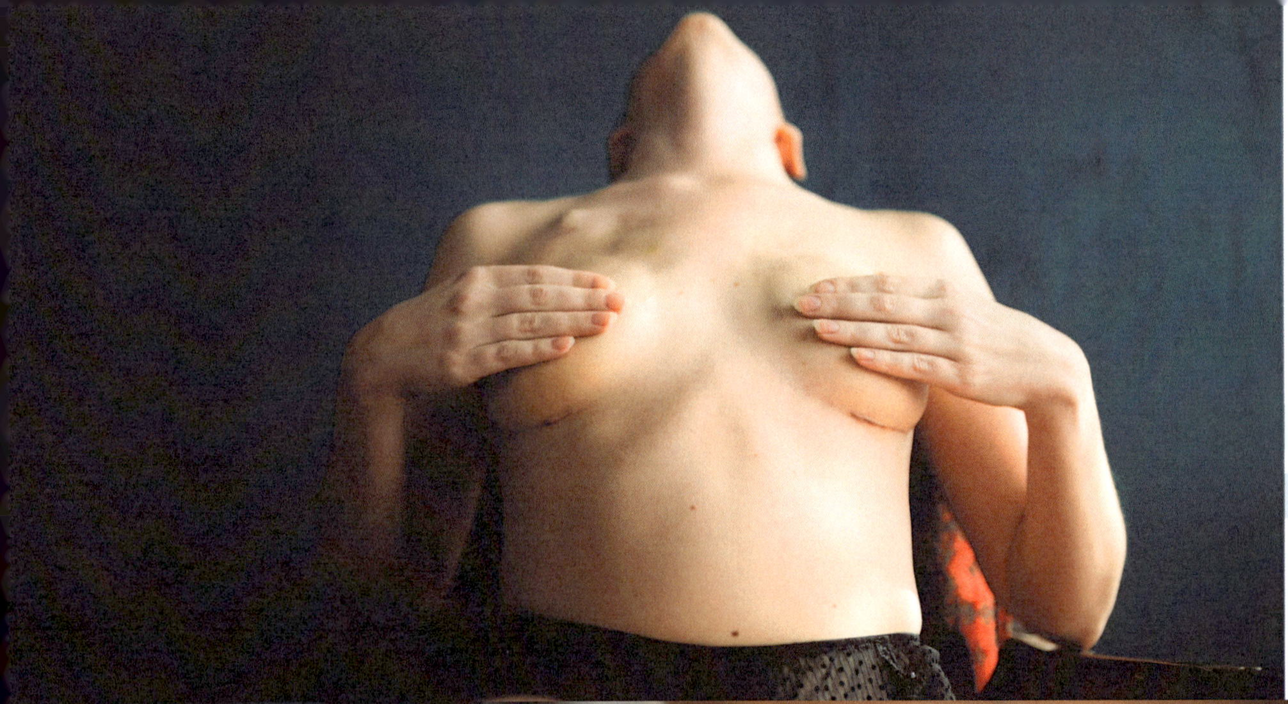
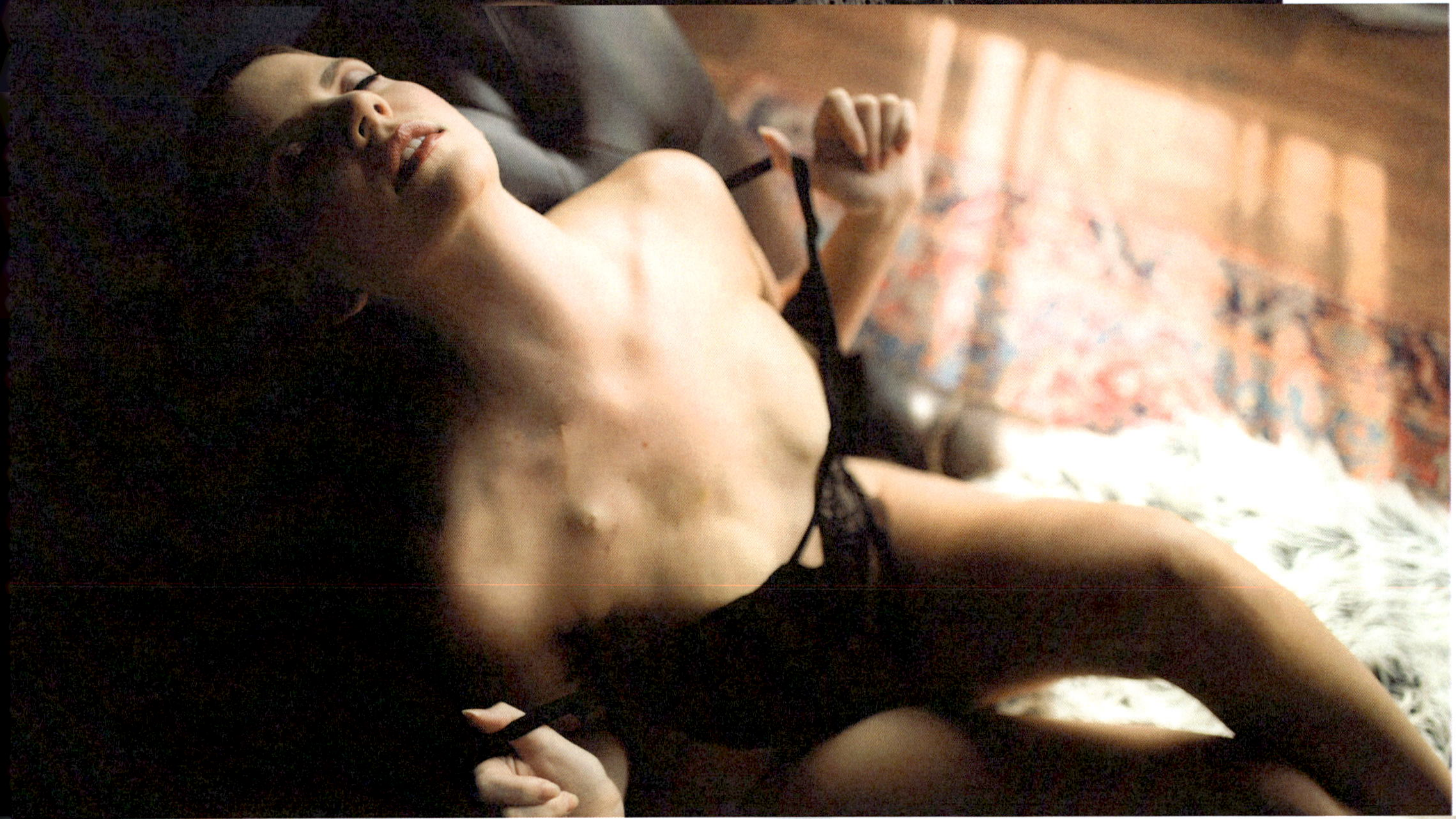
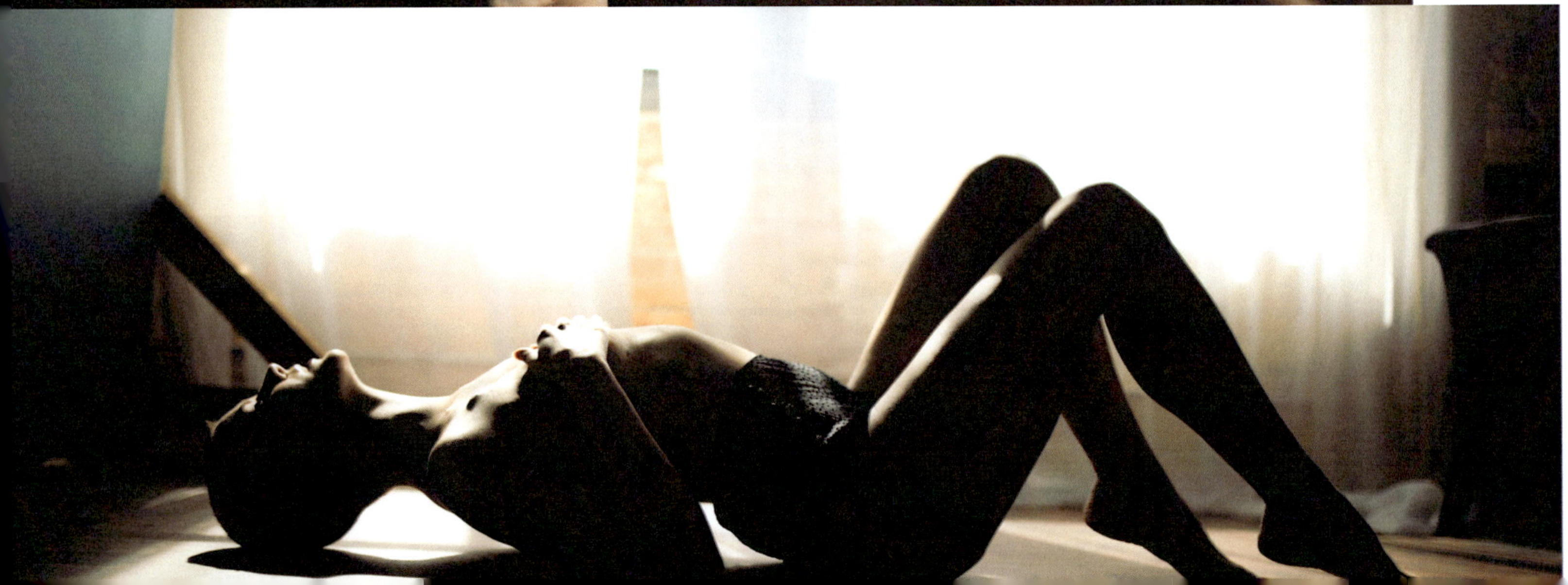

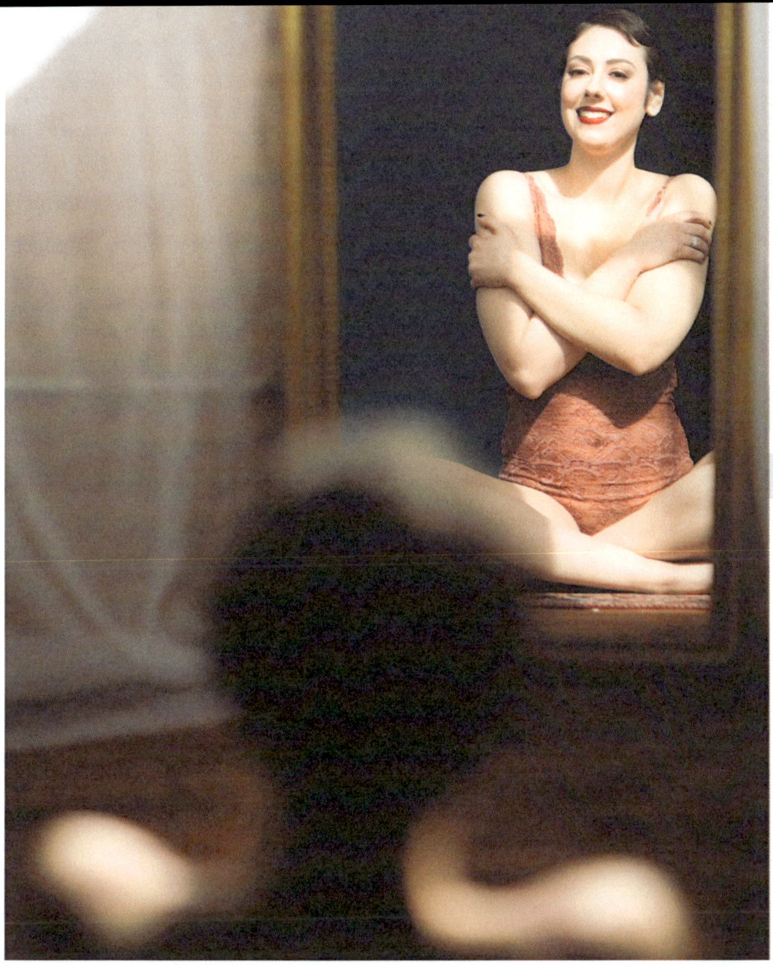

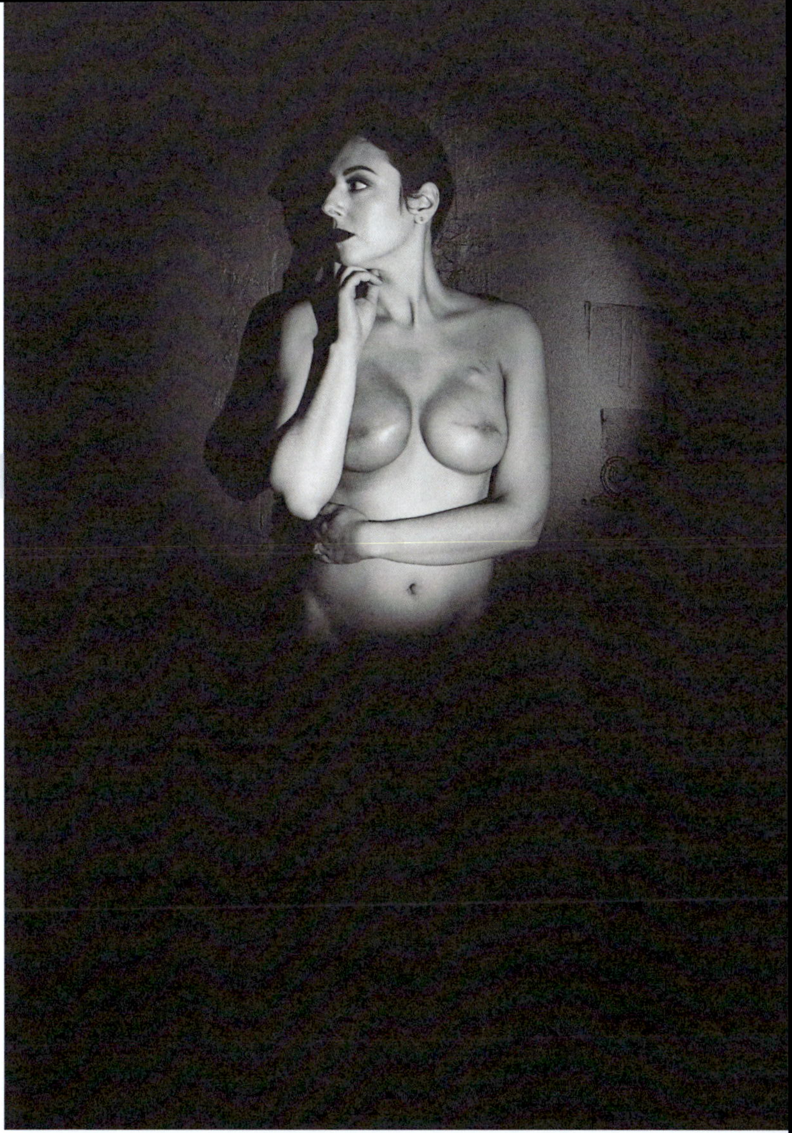

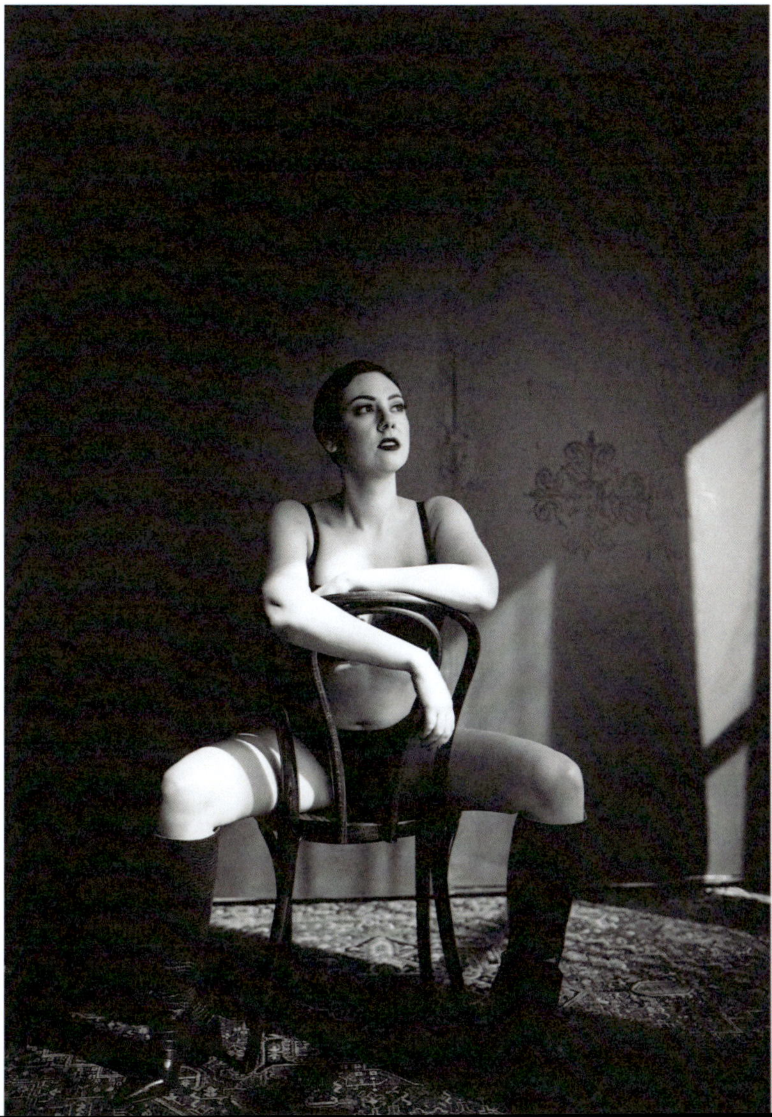

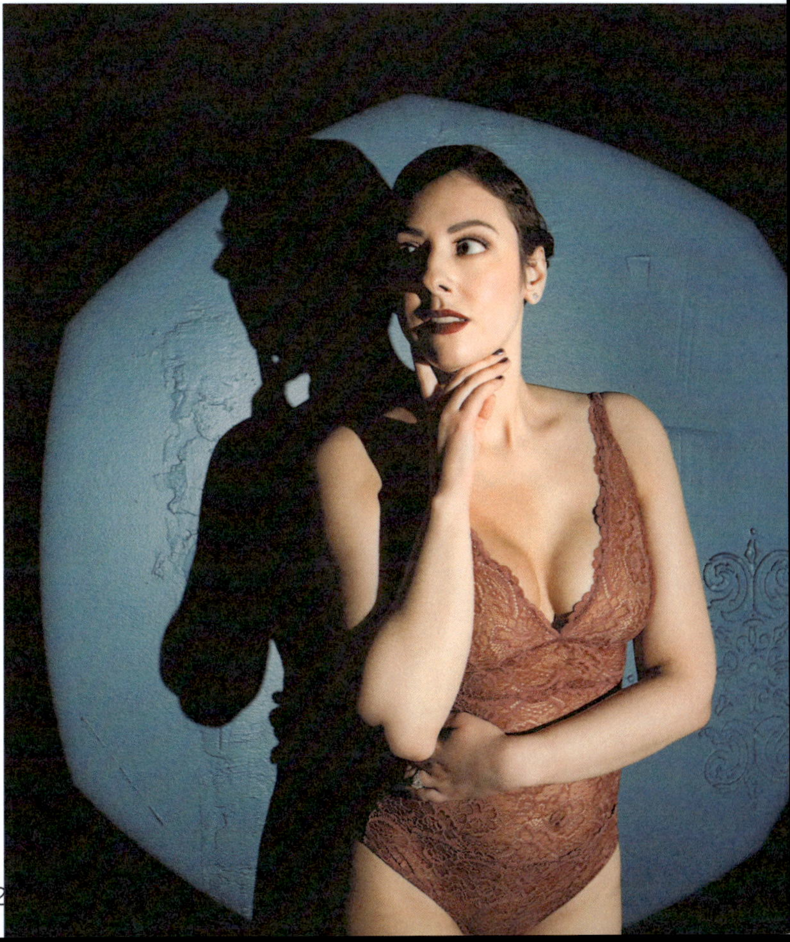

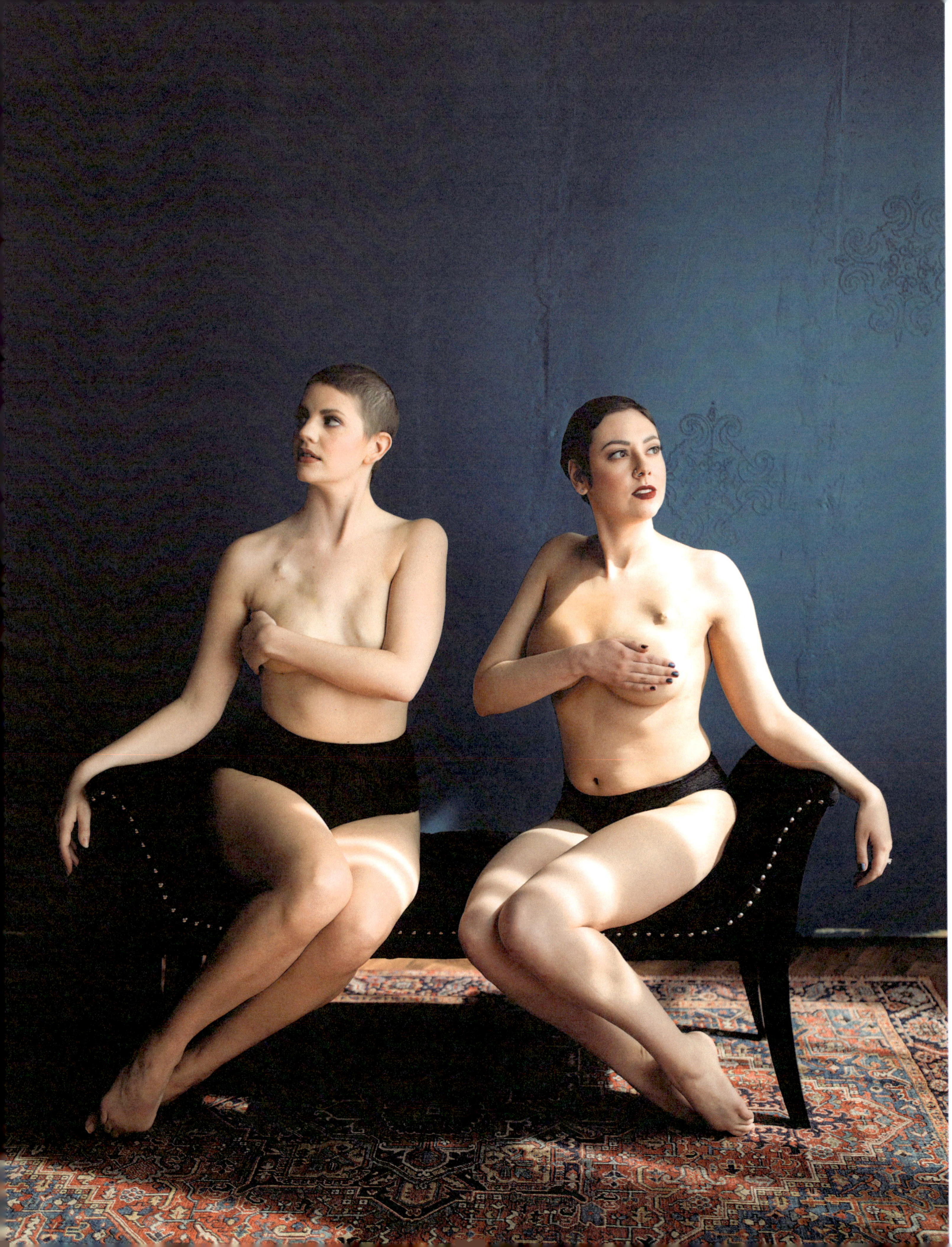

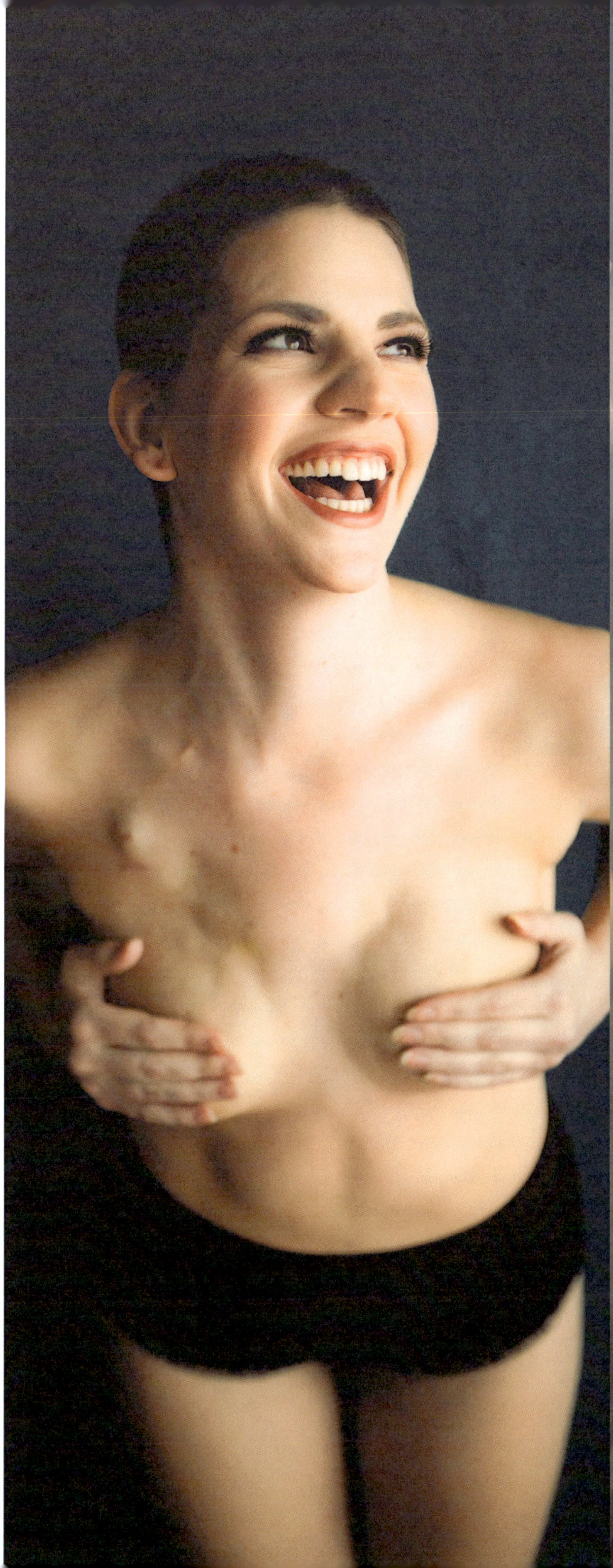

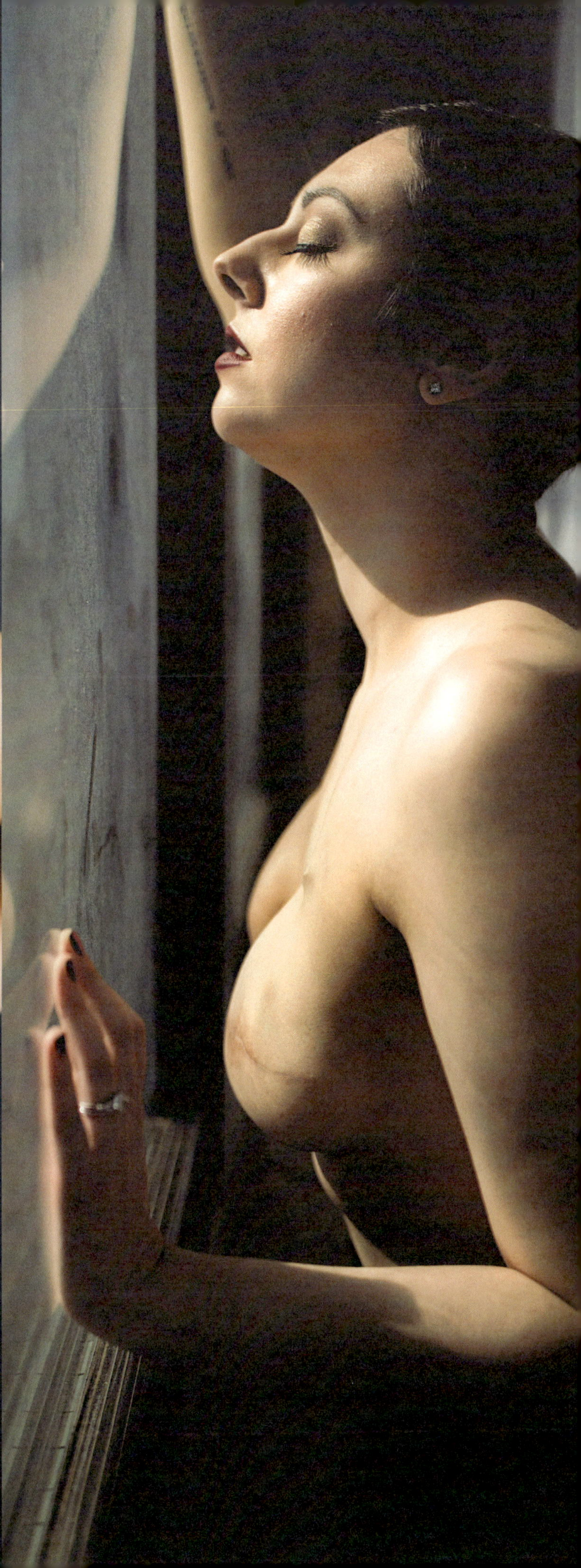

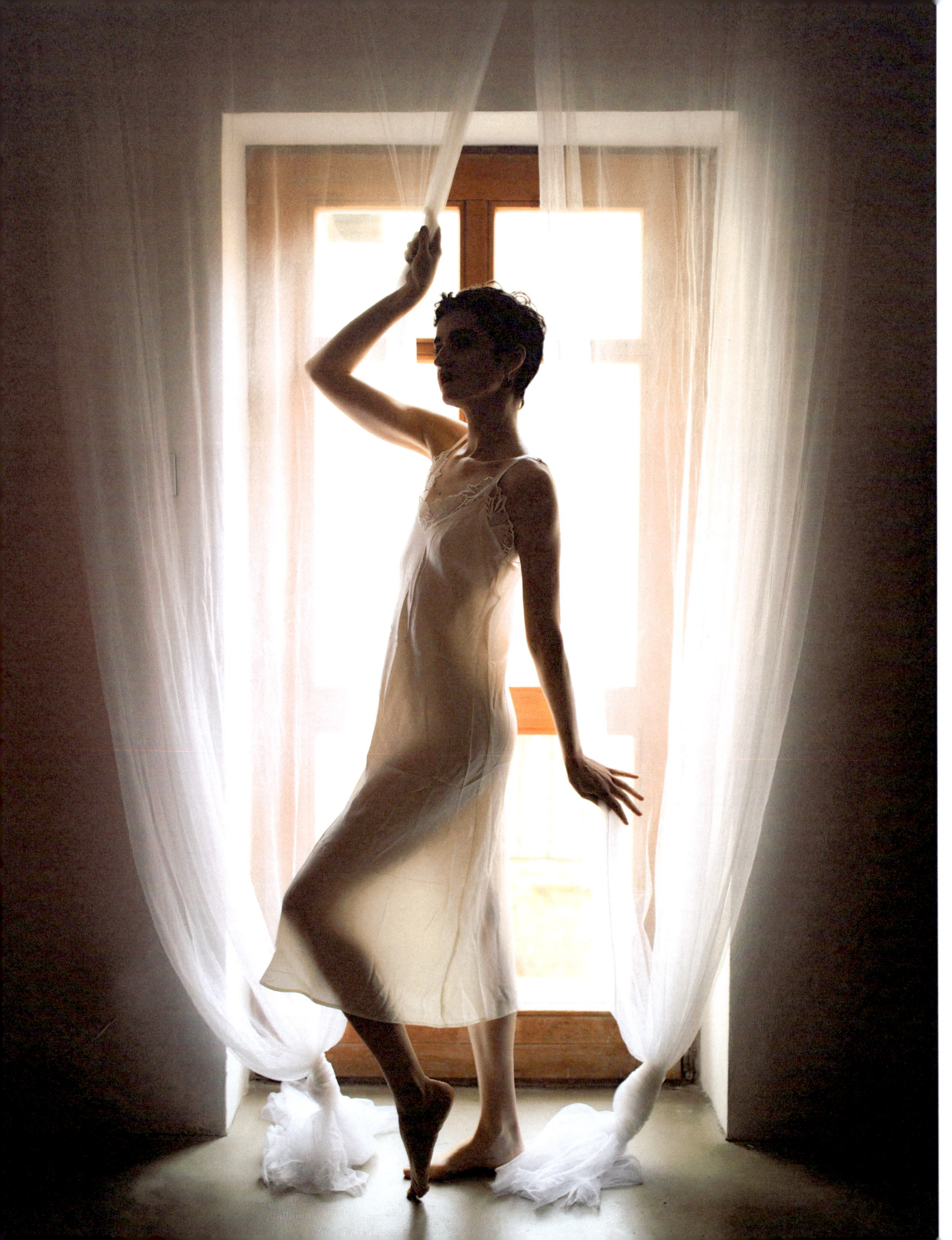

Diagnosis: *Breast Cancer.*
Age Diagnosed: *33 and 34*
Treatments Received: *Surgery, Chemotherapy, Radiation therapy, Anti-hormonal therapy (I stopped it).*
Age at time of photographs: *39*
Stage at time of photographs: *Complete remission.*
Region: *The Netherlands*
Social Media: *@anaroxanamusic*
anaroxana.com

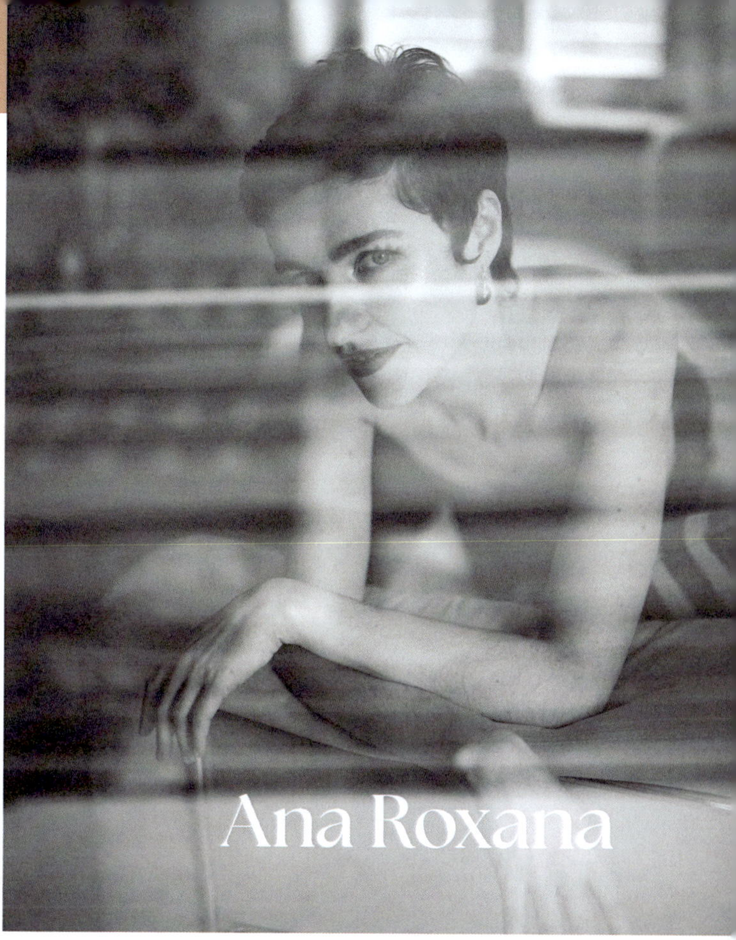

My story

The day after my sister gave birth to my niece in Romania, I learned that I had breast cancer for the second time. It was exactly how life is: good and bad things, fear and joy are all close together.

I was very afraid of all the consequences of chemotherapy. I now know that the fear of the unknown sometimes makes things worse than they are. I had my hair cut short and a hairpiece made of my own hair.

This made the loss of my long beautiful curls more tolerable. And I learned that I am beautiful, with and without hair.

What helped me was repeating to myself often that I am cancer-free. I did this during meditations. It gave me courage and hope that I would be okay.

Breast cancer did not make me feel less of a woman. I even wrote a song One Breast Woman about it. But what I encountered most difficult is how my sex life was impacted.

It seems that many women are passive in the healing process. So my advice is be actively involved in any healing you are undergoing and believe it can heal.

This whole experience made me look different at sexuality, intimacy and also at what I want and need in a partner.

Most important is to know yourself, speak and ask for what you need and if a man's ego is in the way then he is not the right man for you.

The biggest gift I received from the breast cancer experience was getting back to composing songs (which I hadn't done since university). I really did some soul searching during the treatments. For me, making music is not a rational process, it is more of a spiritual/flow process. Being able to sing my own songs and shape them as in my head was very healing and this is my first purpose.

Sharing is the second purpose and I hope that I can bring light and healing to others through my music

I have changed for the better. I embrace myself. This experience made me live more in the present moment, live more in a state of flow, be less perfectionistic and do things even if they are still in a raw form, because perfectionism prevents us from living our life to fullest.

I speak up what I feel more often and don't let fear of rejection swallow my words. Just be yourself and the right choices will be made, and the right people will surround you, and there will be ease.

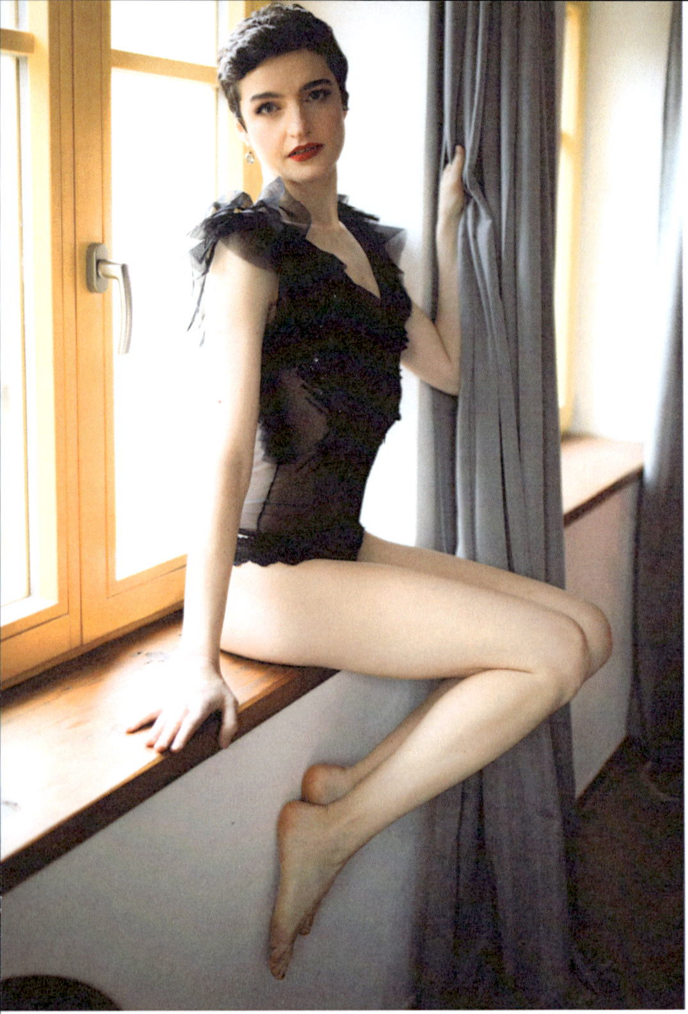
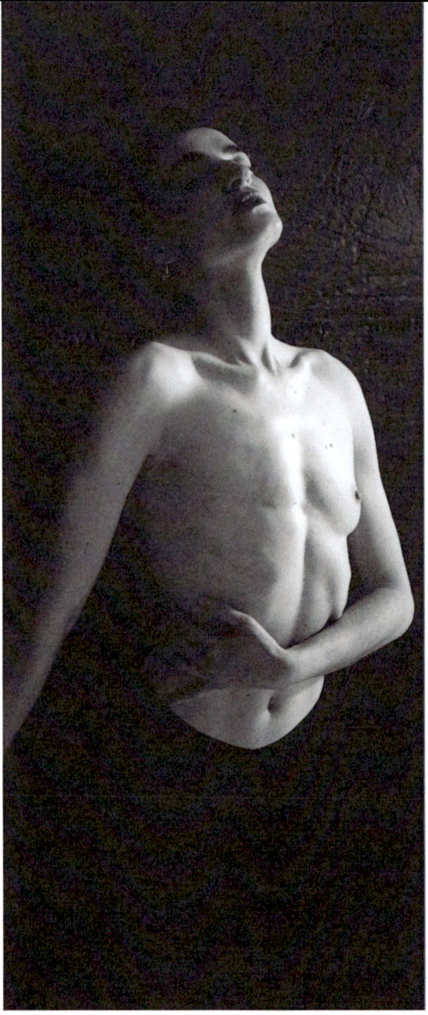
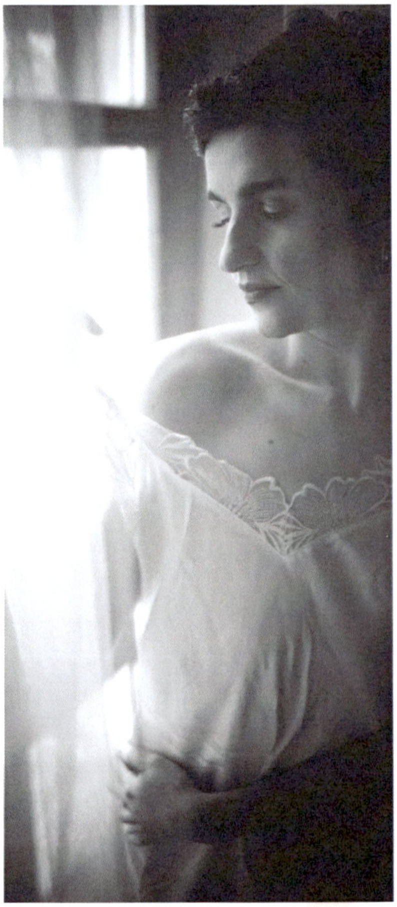
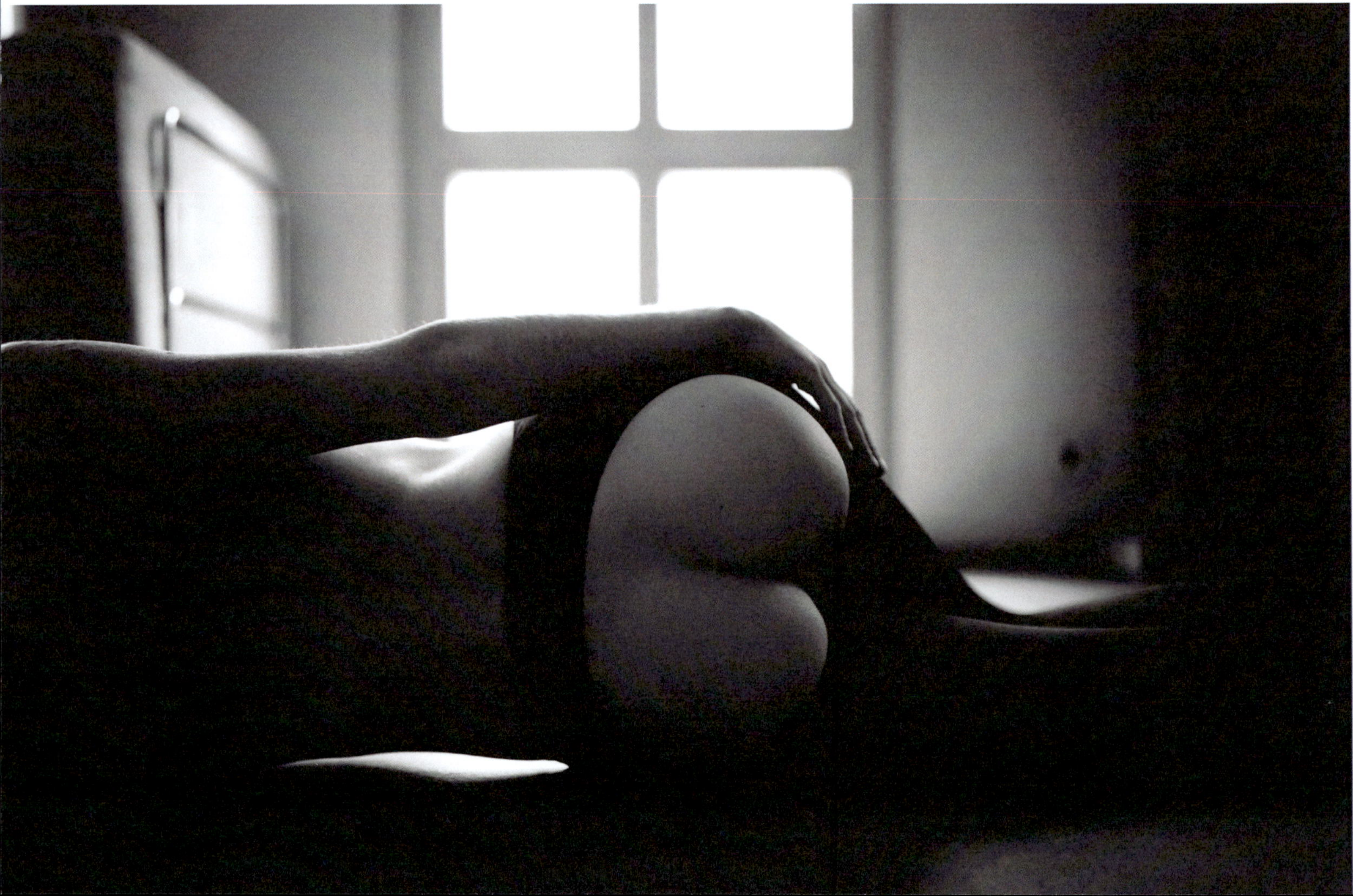

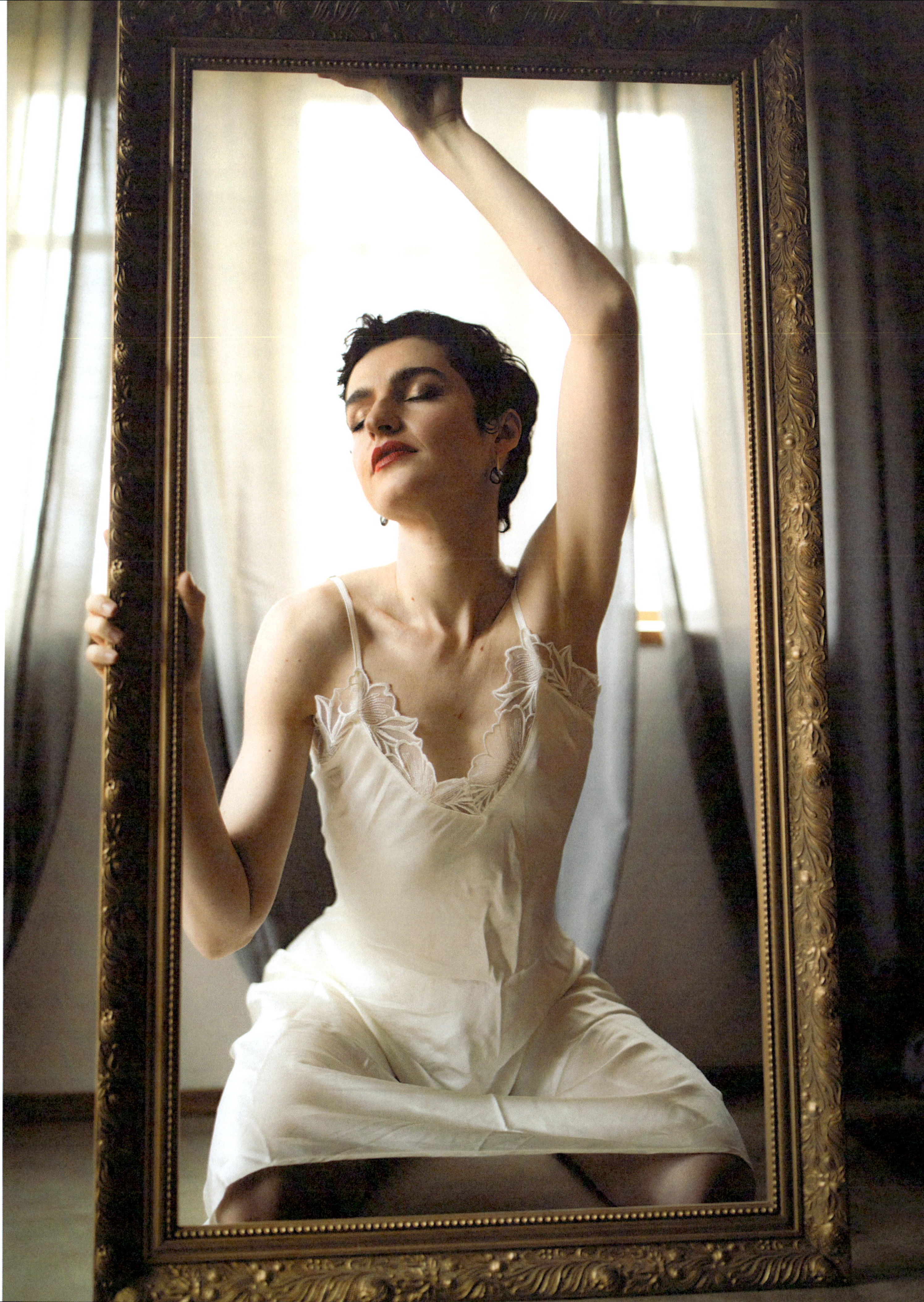

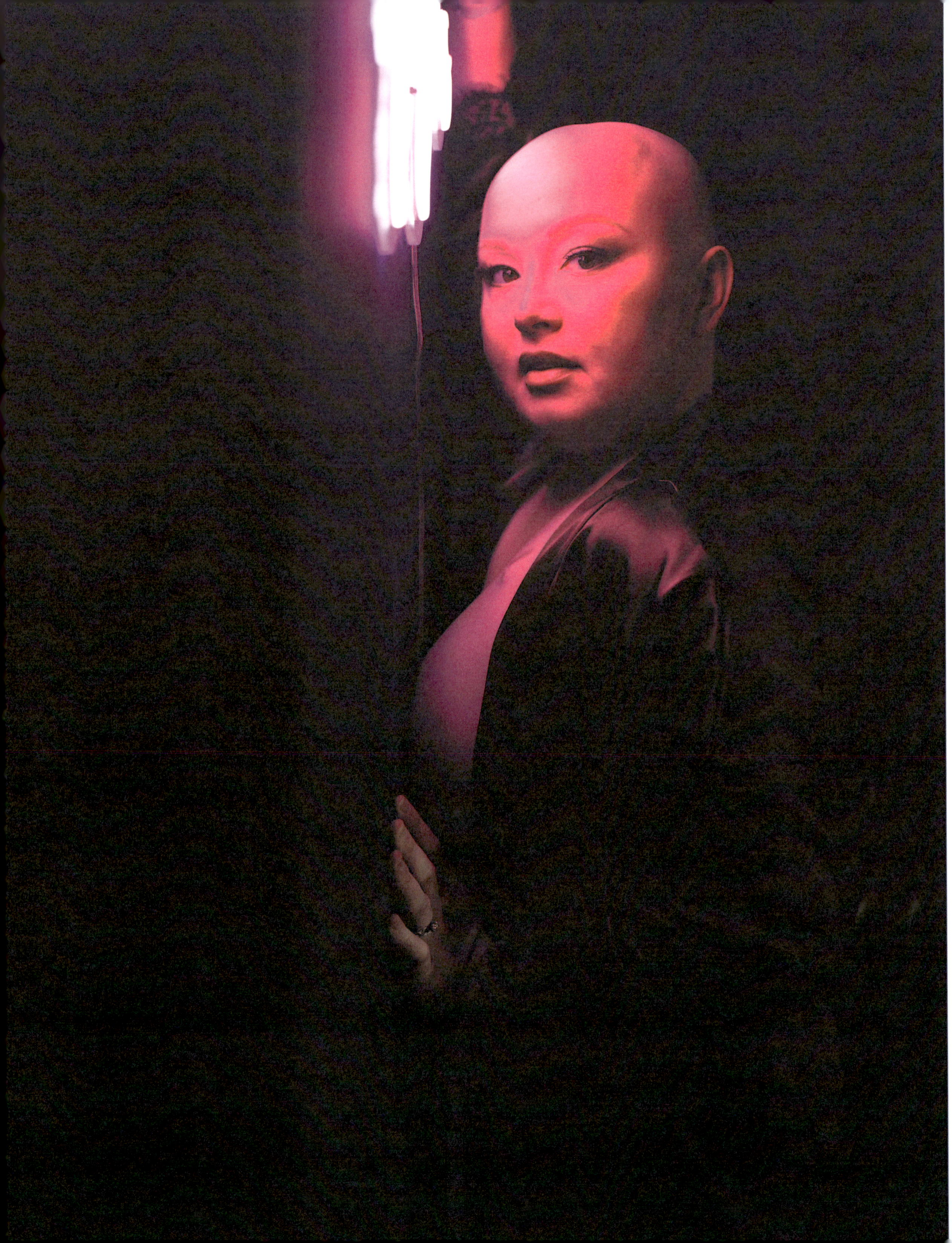

Diagnosis: *Invasive Ductal Carcinoma, Estrogen and Progesterone +, HER2 -*
Age Diagnosed: *31*
Treatments Received: *Right total mastectomy without reconstruction, Chemotherapy, Radiation, Hormonal Therapy, Egg retrieval for fertility preservation.*
Age at time of photographs: *31*
Stage at time of photographs: *After surgery and chemotherapy.*
Region: *New York State*

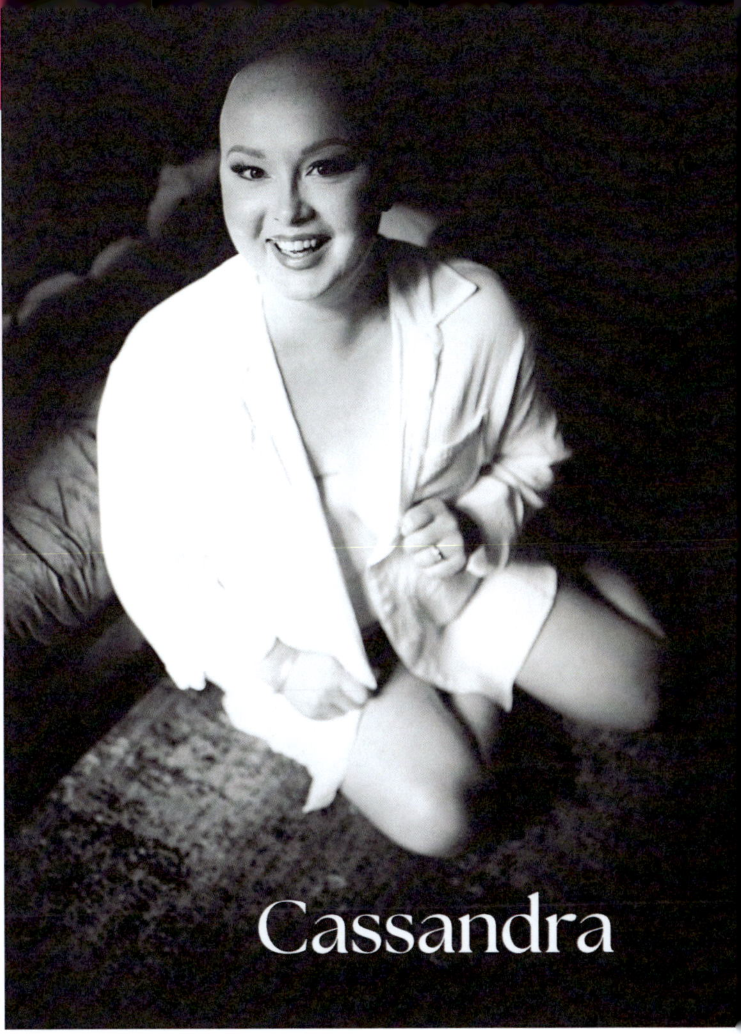

Cassandra

When I got my diagnosis

I was told I had to stop breastfeeding cold turkey before I could have my mastectomy to decrease the risk of post-operative infection.

For a long time, all I could see when looking at my asymmetric chest was the premature loss of that relationship with my son and it made me so angry and sad.

It took months for me to be able to see my scars as proof of my resilience, and to accept that it is okay to be angry about what cancer took from me while also be so thankful and appreciative that I am still here to watch my son grow up.

(He is still a Mommy's Boy, even though I have one less boob.)

I was so terrified of losing my hair, not because I was worried about how I would look, but because I was worried about how my 2-year-old son would react when my hair fell out.

I couldn't stomach the idea of my toddler being scared of mommy without hair.

The day that I decided to shave my head because I couldn't handle it slowly falling out anymore, I was so nervous for him to come home from daycare.

But he ran in the door, hugged me and laughed saying that I matched daddy now (who is also bald).

He then asked to match too and we buzzed his hair for the first time.

I realized that my hair didn't define me or my role as his mom and started to embrace my bald head.

I often chose to go out in public without a head covering or wig and felt that my bald head was a sign of my strength and perseverance.

Now my hair has grown back in the most beautiful ringlet curls that have stuck around 2 years later and remind me every day that I am stronger than I ever thought I would have to be.

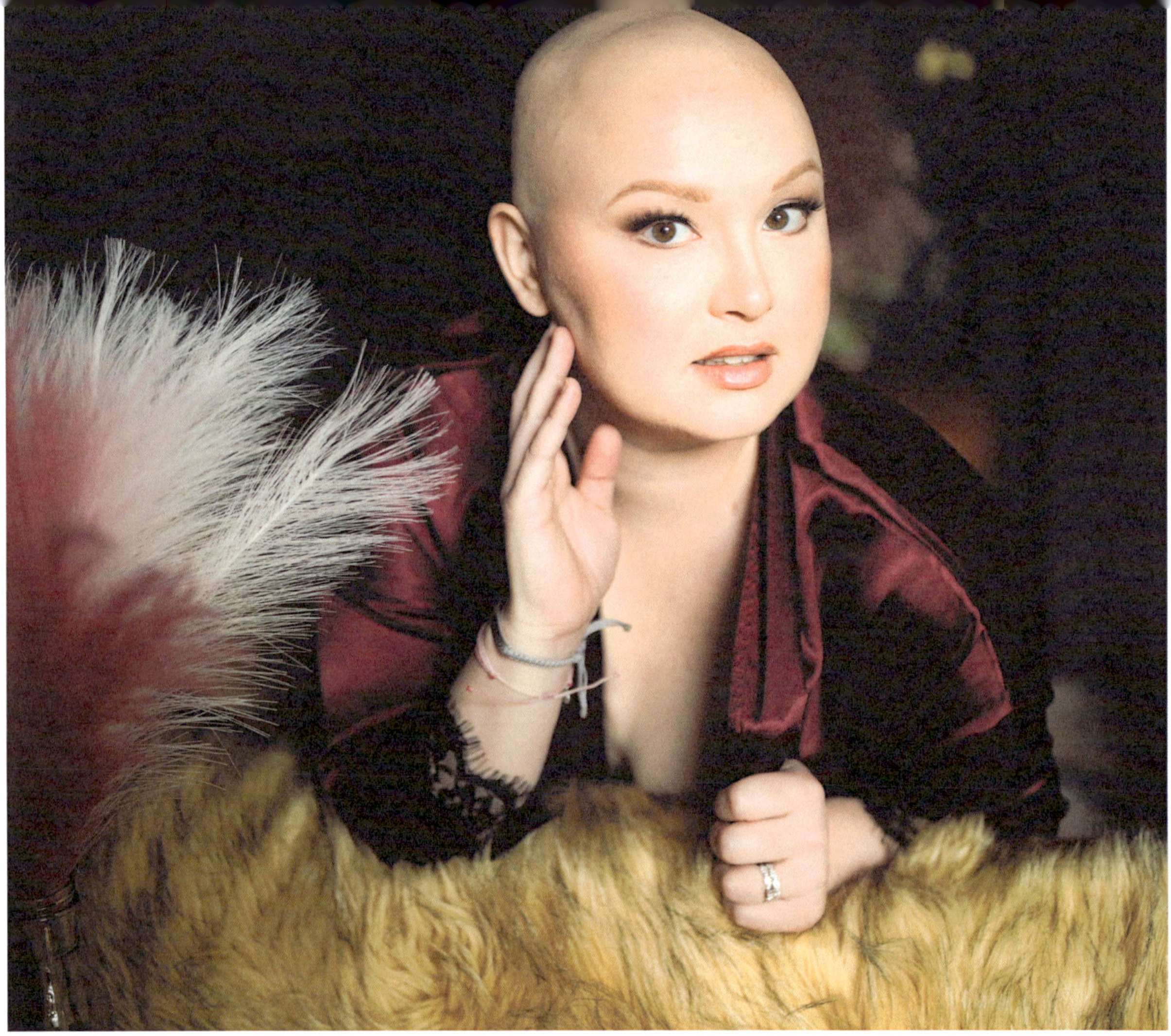

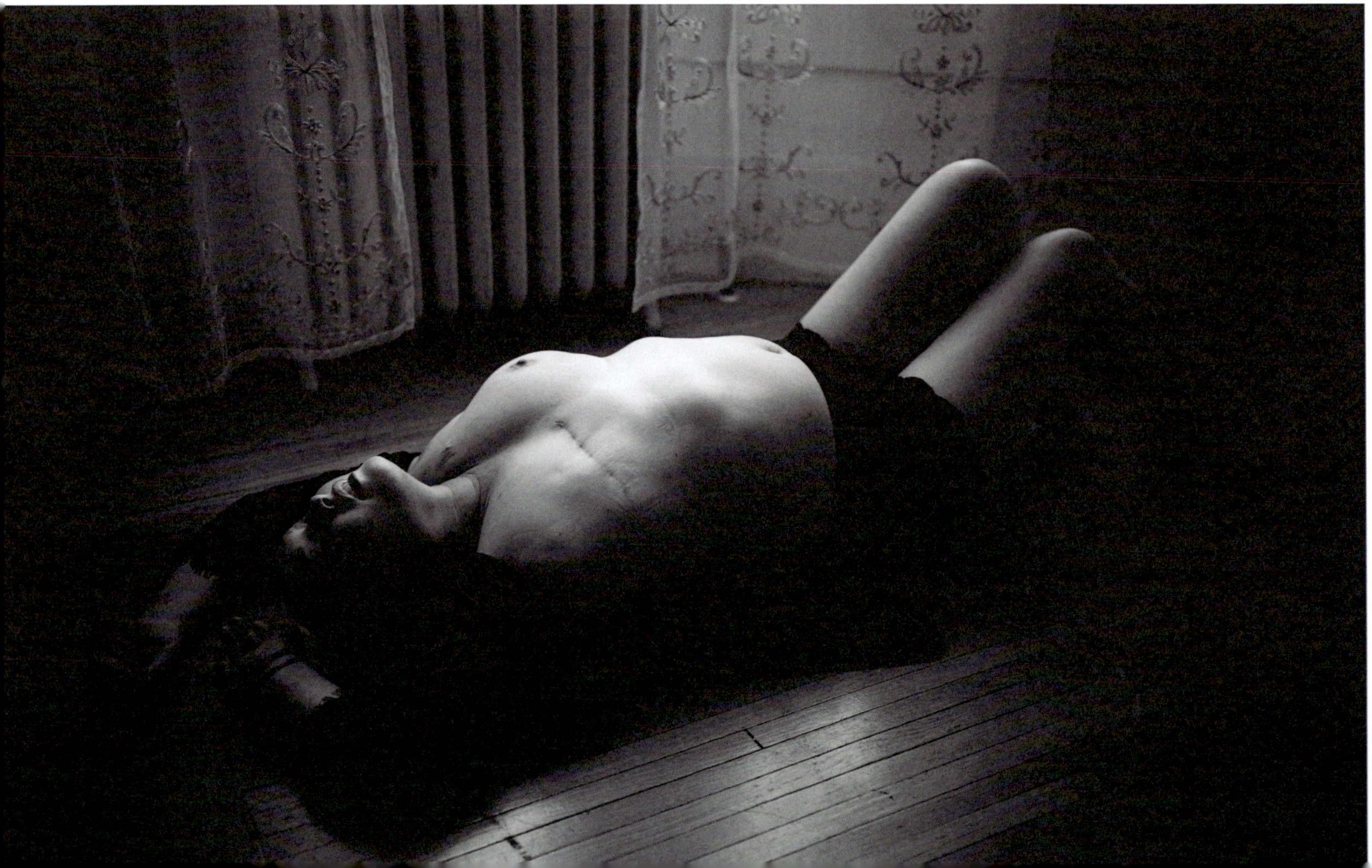

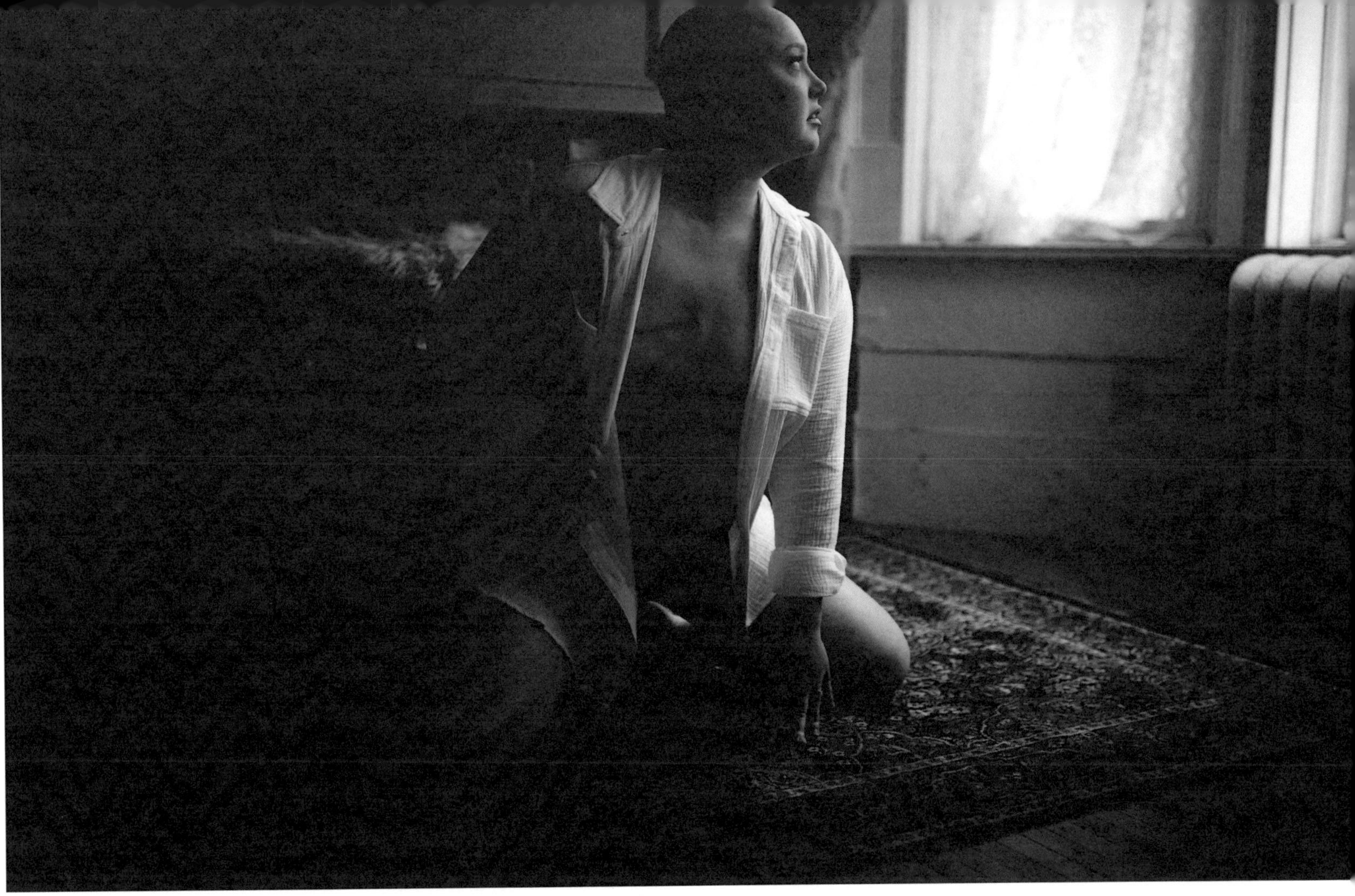

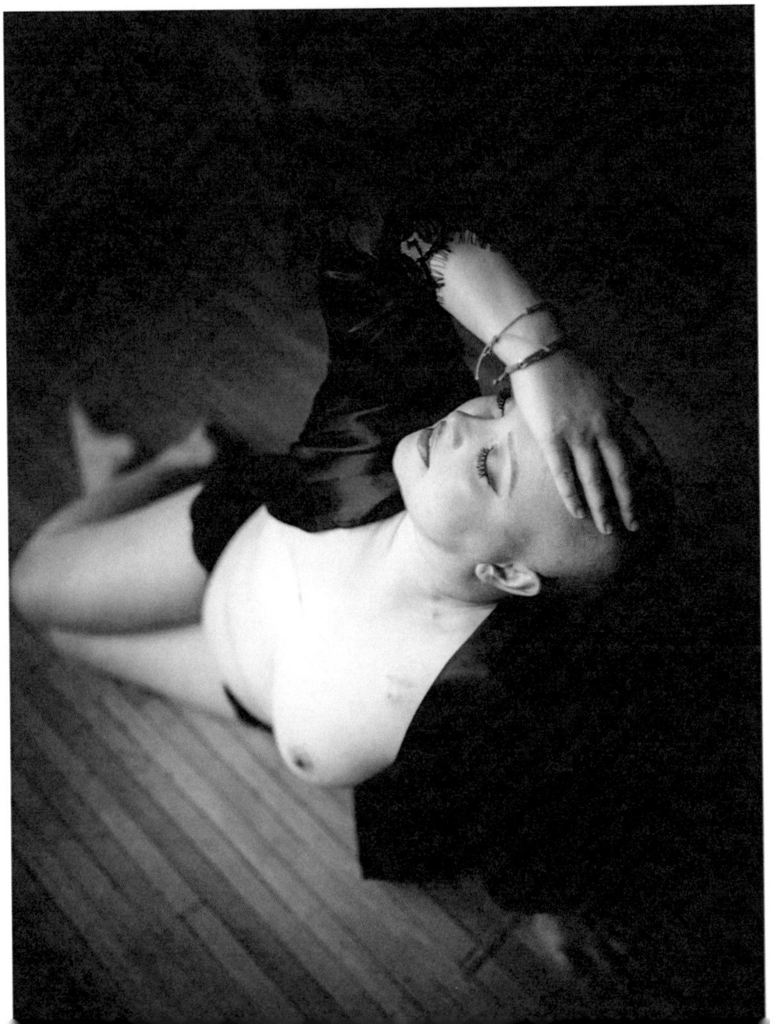

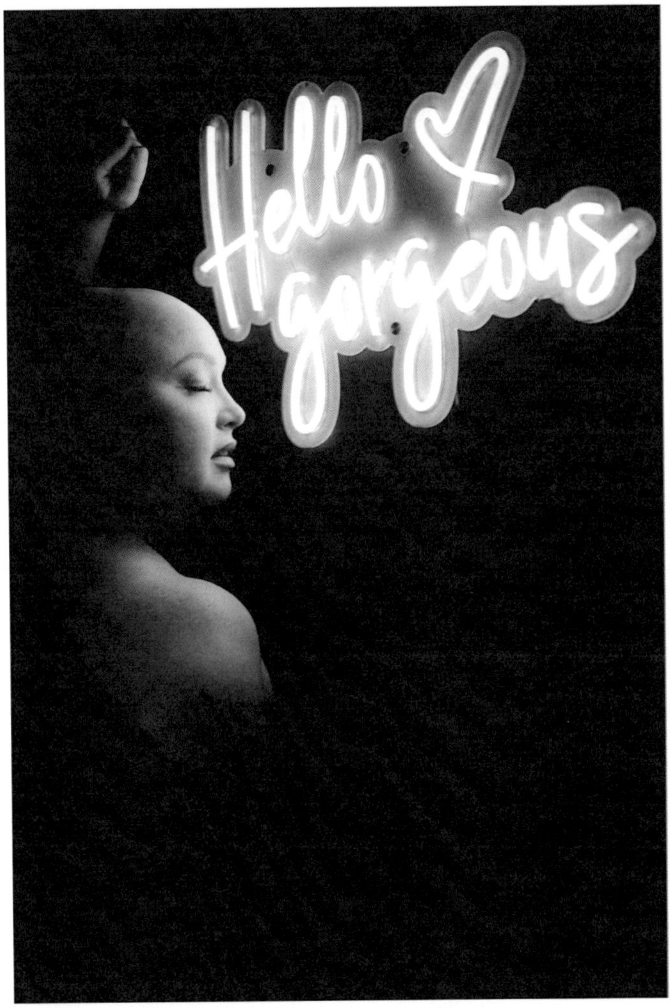
Hello gorgeous

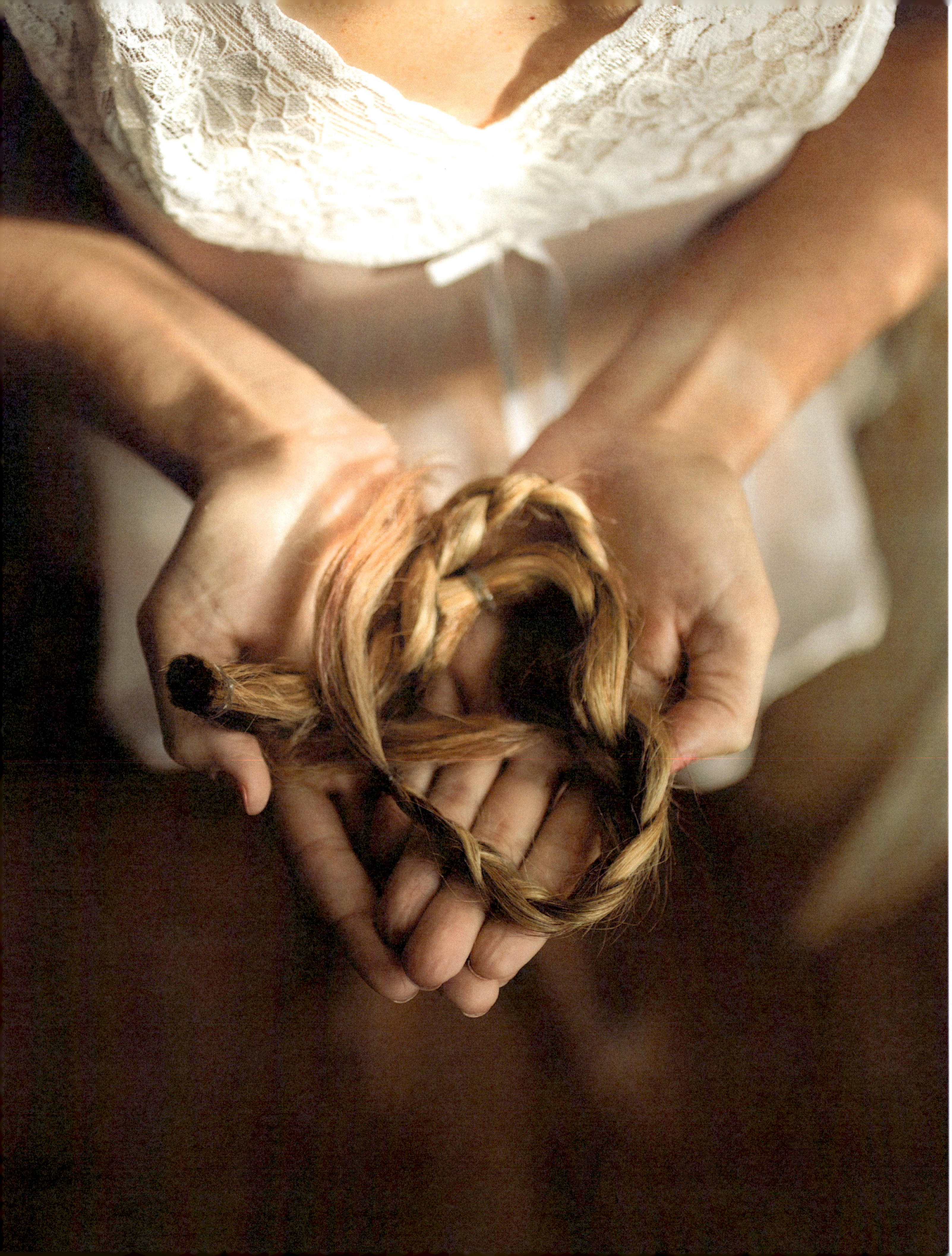

Erin

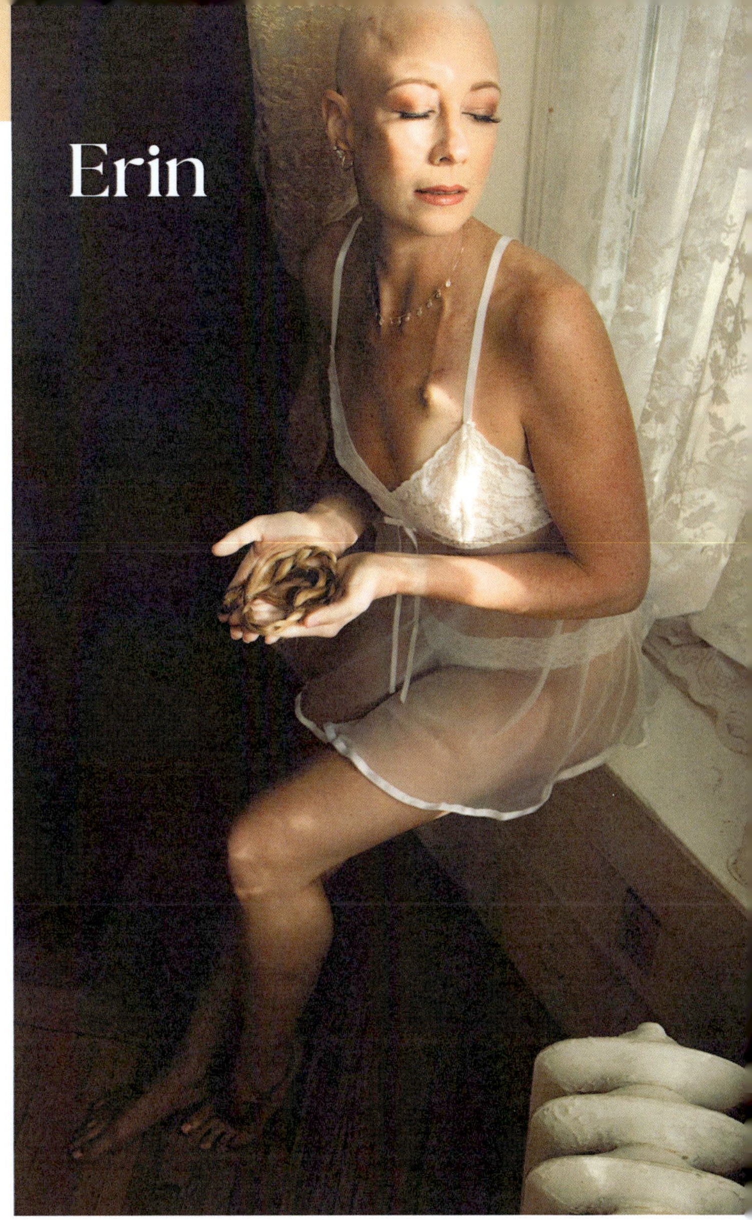

Diagnosis: *Breast cancer, ER/PR/HER2 triple positive.*
Age Diagnosed: *44*
Treatments Received: *2 rounds of chemotherapy, 28 days of radiation, bi-lateral mastectomy.*
Age at time of photographs: *44*
Stage at time of photographs: *Stage 1*
Region: *United States*

Before being diagnosed with cancer

I felt like I was on top of the world, having landed a new job.

I was on a new workout regimen as health was a priority for me.

During treatment, my health diminished quickly, however, I was grateful for how fast my body seemed to heal itself in between chemotherapy sessions.

I tried to remain active, but there were days it took all of me just to move a couple of feet from one room to the other or to get downstairs.

I gave myself the grace I needed and leaned on my tribe to help lift me up.

Since I recently finished up my second round of chemotherapy, I can see my body changing in positive ways and I am thrilled to be able to put the work in to rebuild my body to a healthy state.Confidence comes from inside of every one of us.

It is hard to see our health and body deteriorate through this journey but for me I kept sight of the light at the end of the tunnel.

Knowing that there would be an end, gave me hope that I could and will get back to the best me possible.
I was able to learn to let things go, and that helped relieve stress and worry.

I kept a light journal to my Facebook family/ friends. It sounds silly, but when I posted, they responded, and it lifted me up in the times when I needed it the most!

This was the biggest eye-opening experience for me, that my true tribe came to my side to lift me up.

I regained friendships that were lost in life somewhere along the line, and I can say 100% that I would go through the journey again knowing that I gained those friendships back.

Don't be afraid, rather respect that this is something you are going to face and that you will overcome it!

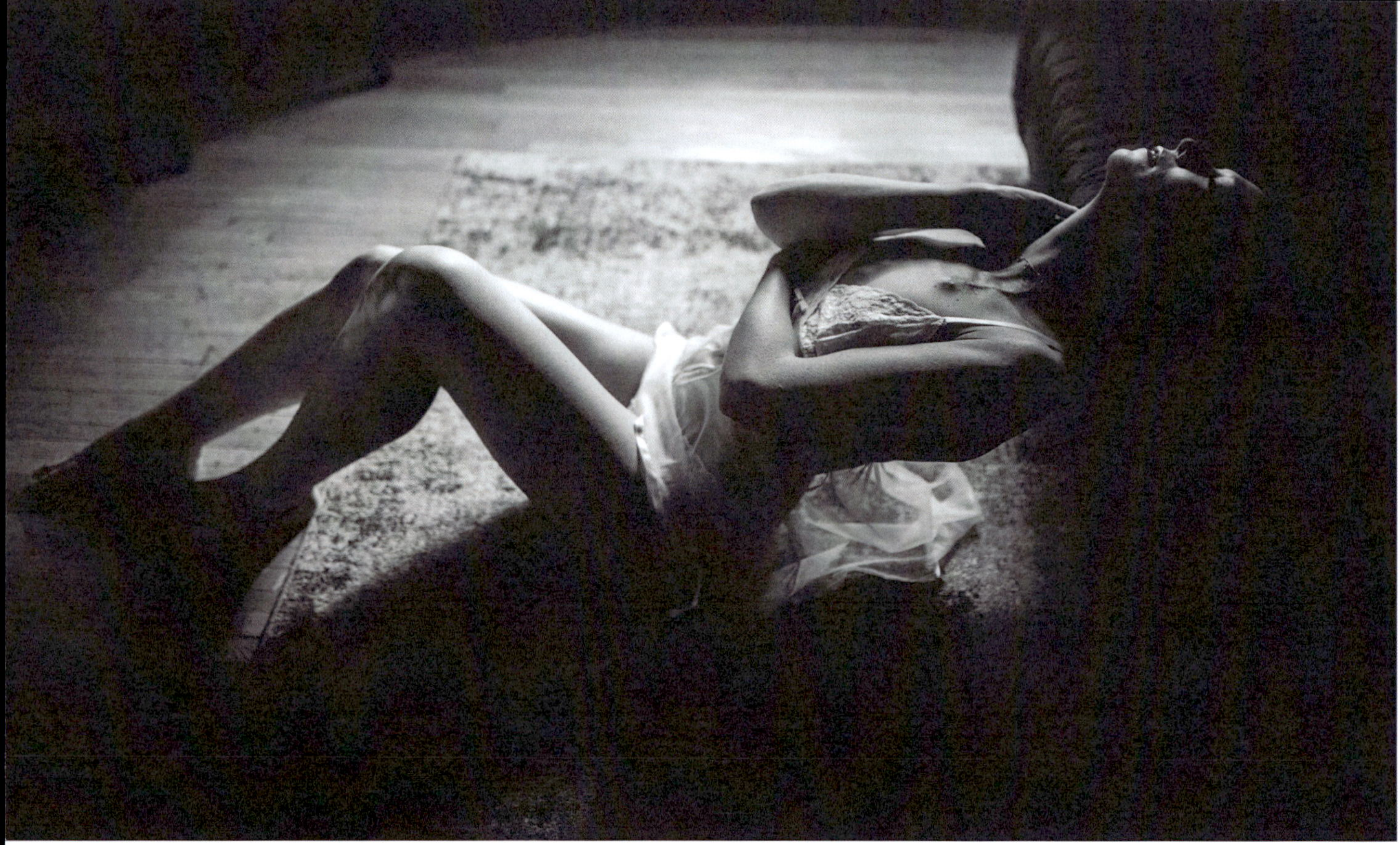
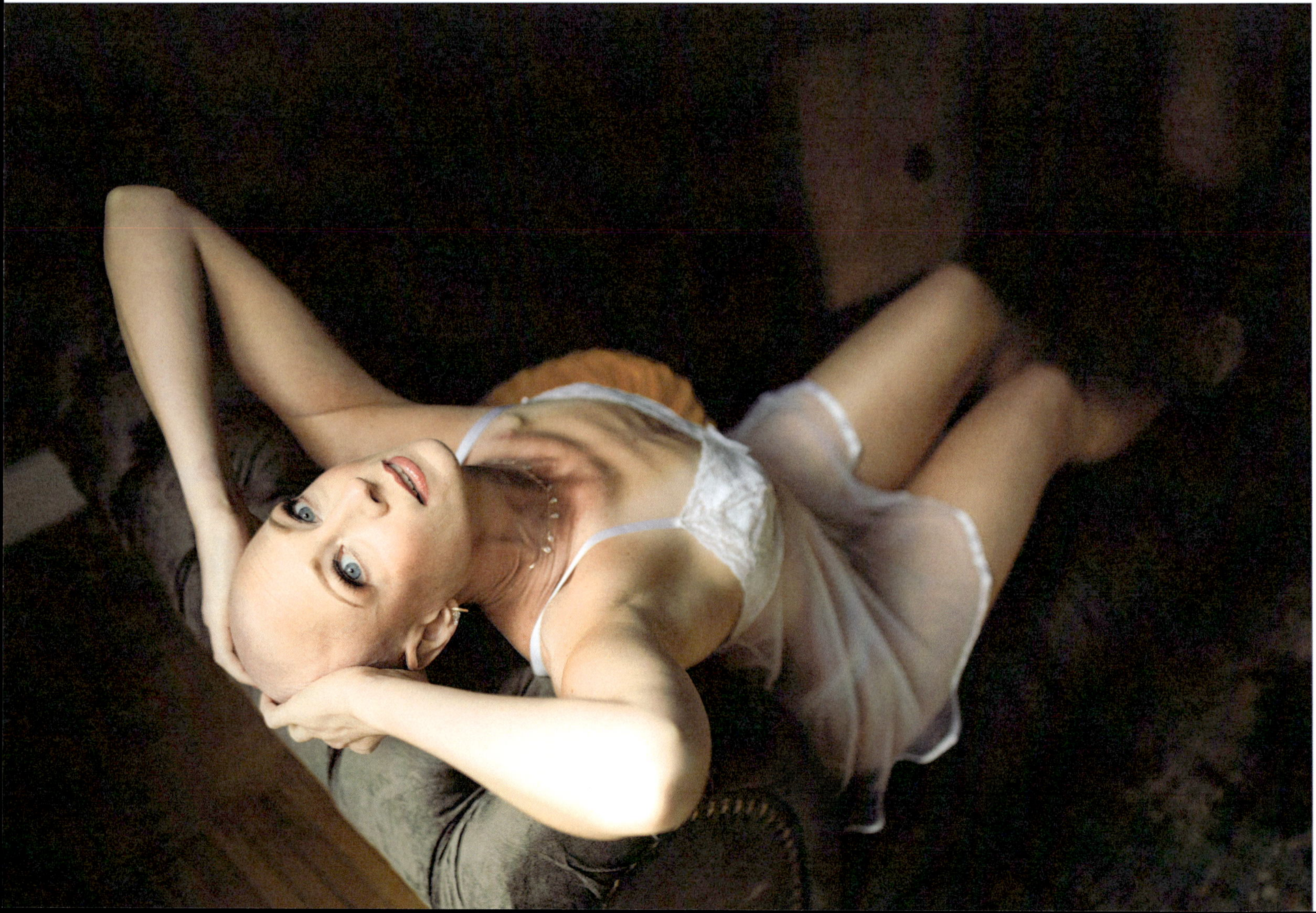

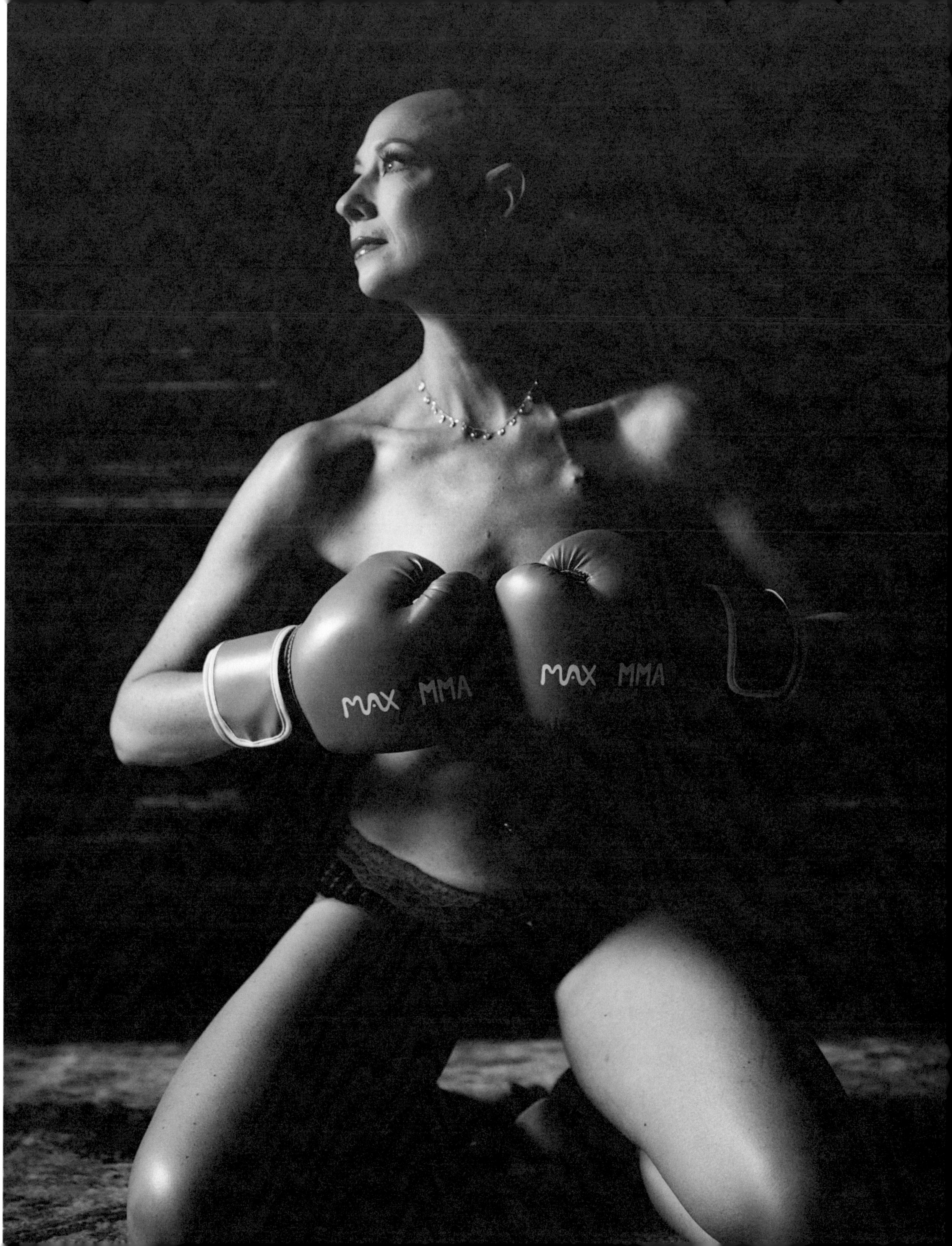
MAX MMA
MAX MMA

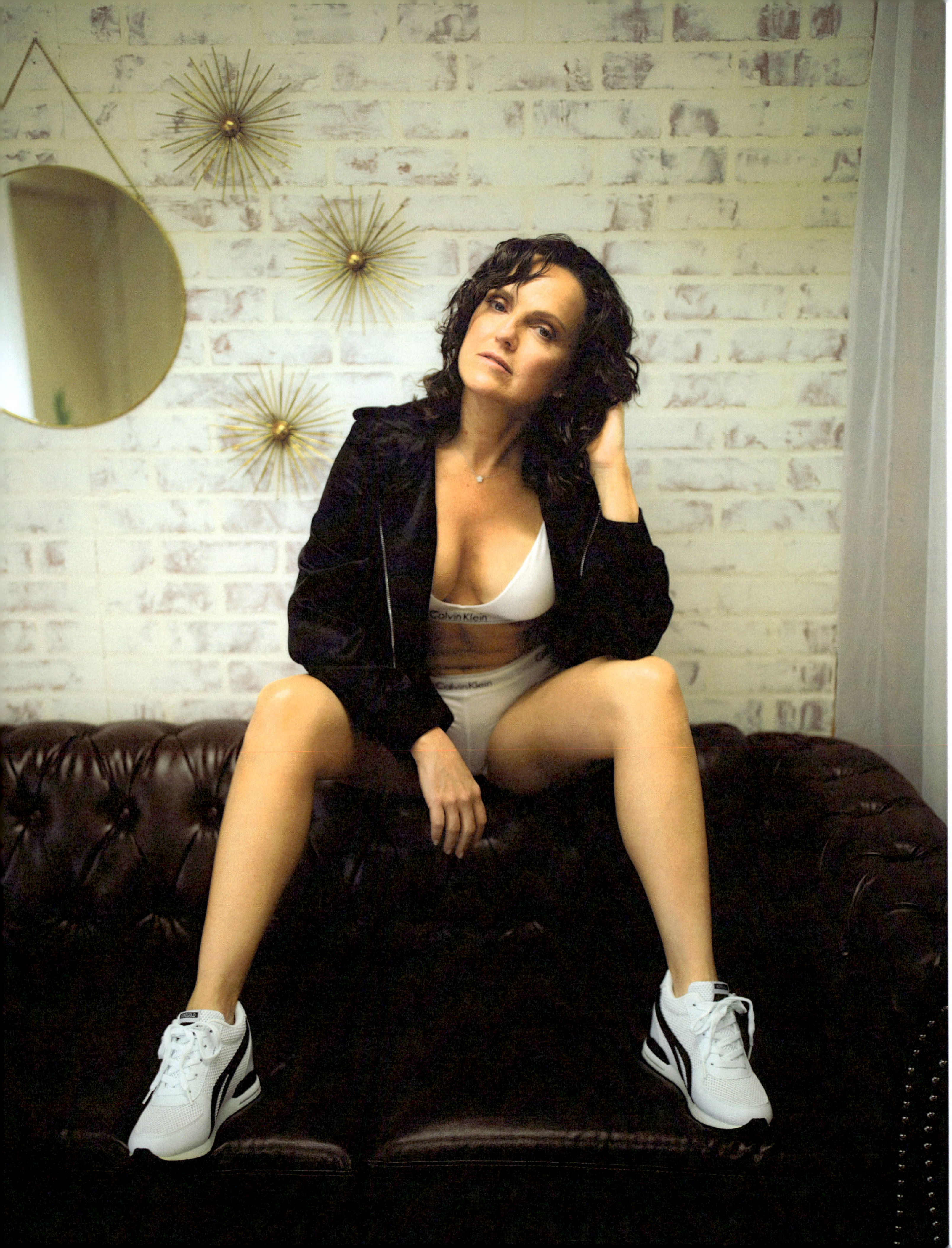
Calvin Klein
Calvin Klein

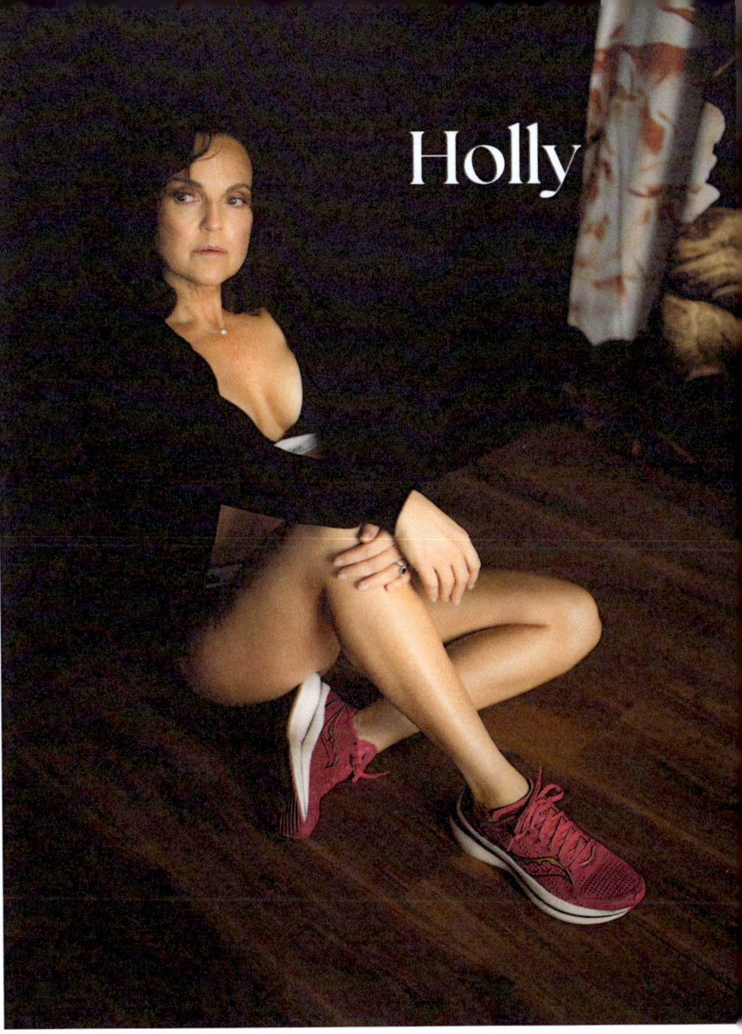

Diagnosis: *Stage 3 HER2+ Invasive Ductal Carcinoma.*
Age Diagnosed: *51*
Treatments Received: *Chemotherapy, Bilateral Mastectomy, Radiation.*
Age at time of photographs: *53*
Stage at time of photographs: *Treatment Completed, Cancer Free.*
Region: *Colorado*

Before cancer

I said a lot of horrible things to my body. I was so critical of every tiny detail and obsessed over every part of it. I did take care of my body with exercise, running and healthy organic foods, which is why so many people in my circle were shocked that I was the one to get cancer. I had just finished running a marathon a few weeks before my diagnosis. As I went through chemo, surgery and radiation, I started to feel a deep appreciation of what my body was able to do, how it healed itself with every new challenge we threw at it.

With each new scar, I began to speak differently to my body- I had more compassion. I felt deep gratitude. I saw incredible beauty where I used to see flaws. I am back to training again and I marvel at what my body is able to do. I thank my body after every run, every workout and every morning that it is able to rise up out of bed and tackle the challenges of life.

If you aren't happy with something or it doesn't feel right to you, don't settle for whatever that is and tell yourself you have to live with it. After my consultation with the first surgeon about reconstruction, I went home and cried.

The after pictures she showed me were devastating and she was recommending a surgery that would affect the use of my left arm stating that, "it doesn't matter because you aren't left-handed." After the shock of that encounter, I went to my breast surgeon and just told her that I would not work with that doctor for reconstruction. I am so incredibly grateful that I found the strength to advocate for myself because I found another doctor who gave me a less invasive procedure and much better cosmetic result.

I was incredibly self-conscious about my thin hair and my new body. I still had pain everywhere and I never knew how long my energy would last. My face was puffy from the treatment and I had spontaneous nosebleeds that made me wonder when I would have to run to a bathroom at the office. It was completely exhausting.

What helped me during that time was starting to participate in activities that made me feel like myself again. I had brunch with supportive friends. I started working out and running again. I cooked delicious meals with my husband. I traveled to fun familiar places. I worked with a talented therapist who helped me adjust to my new normal.

My pain subsided, the nosebleeds stopped and my confidence gradually came back (along with some very curly hair! 😊).

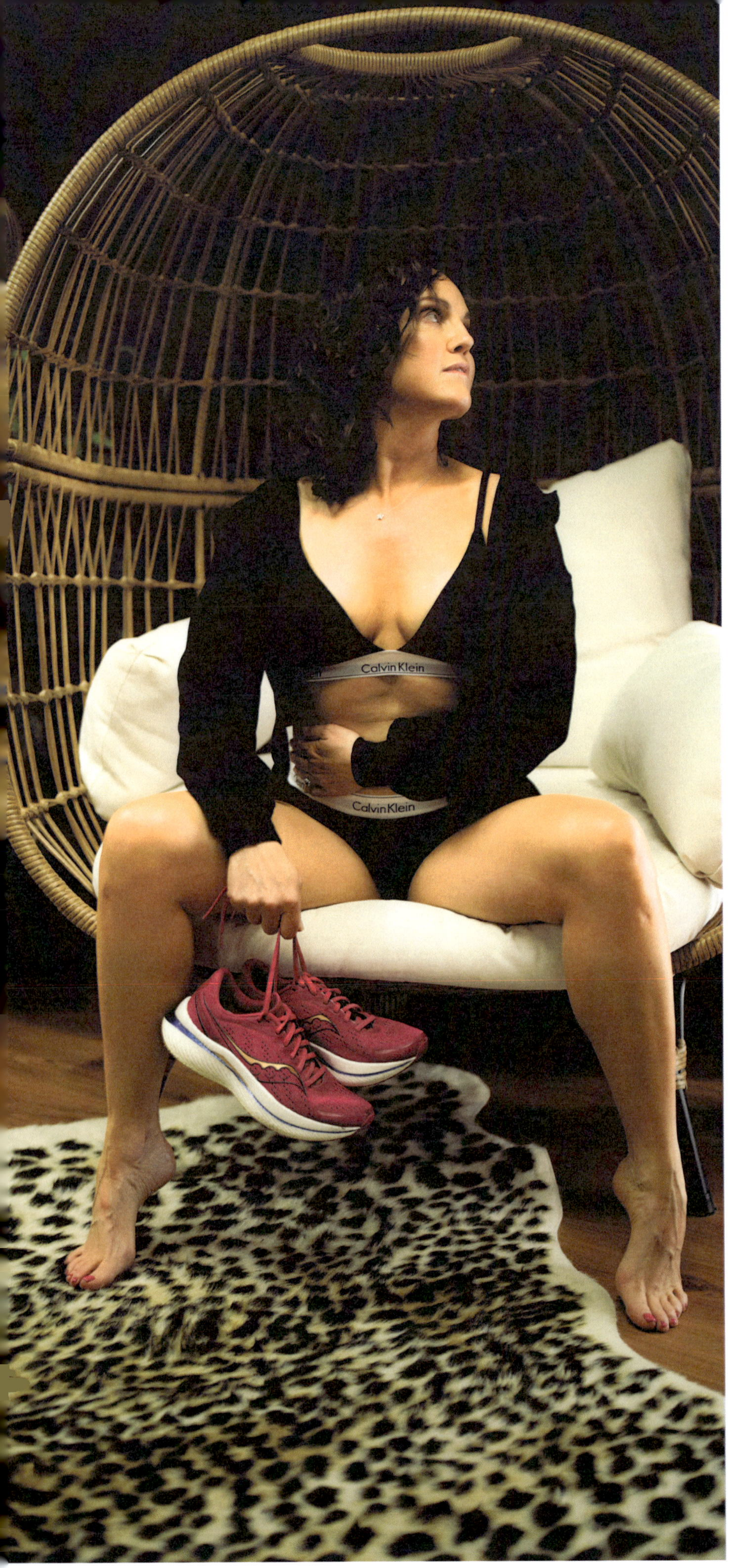
Calvin Klein
Calvin Klein

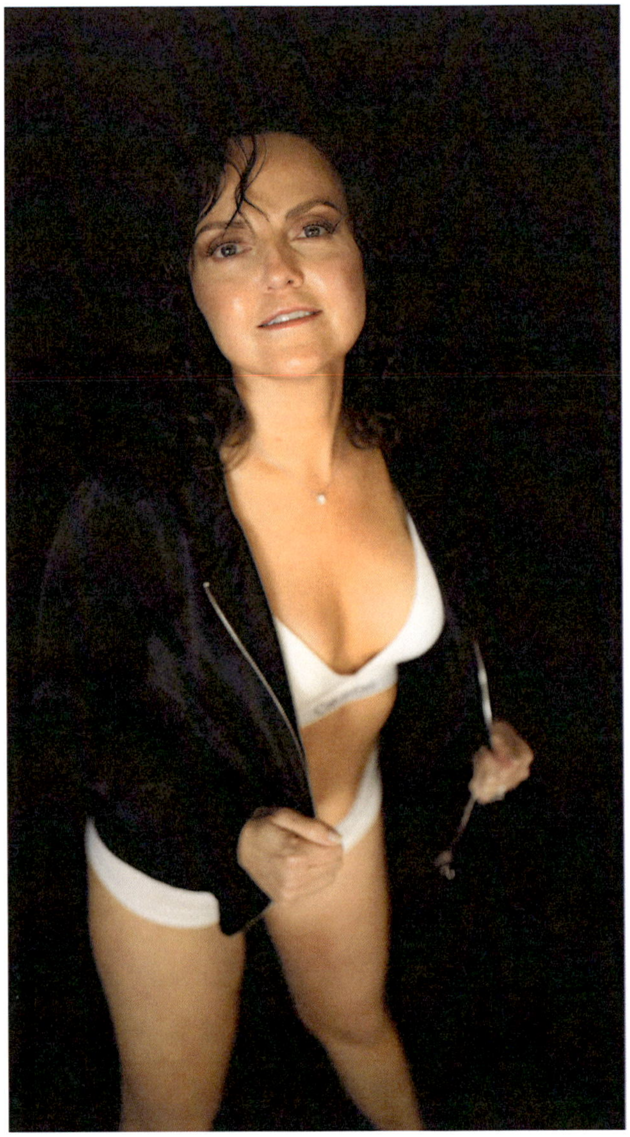

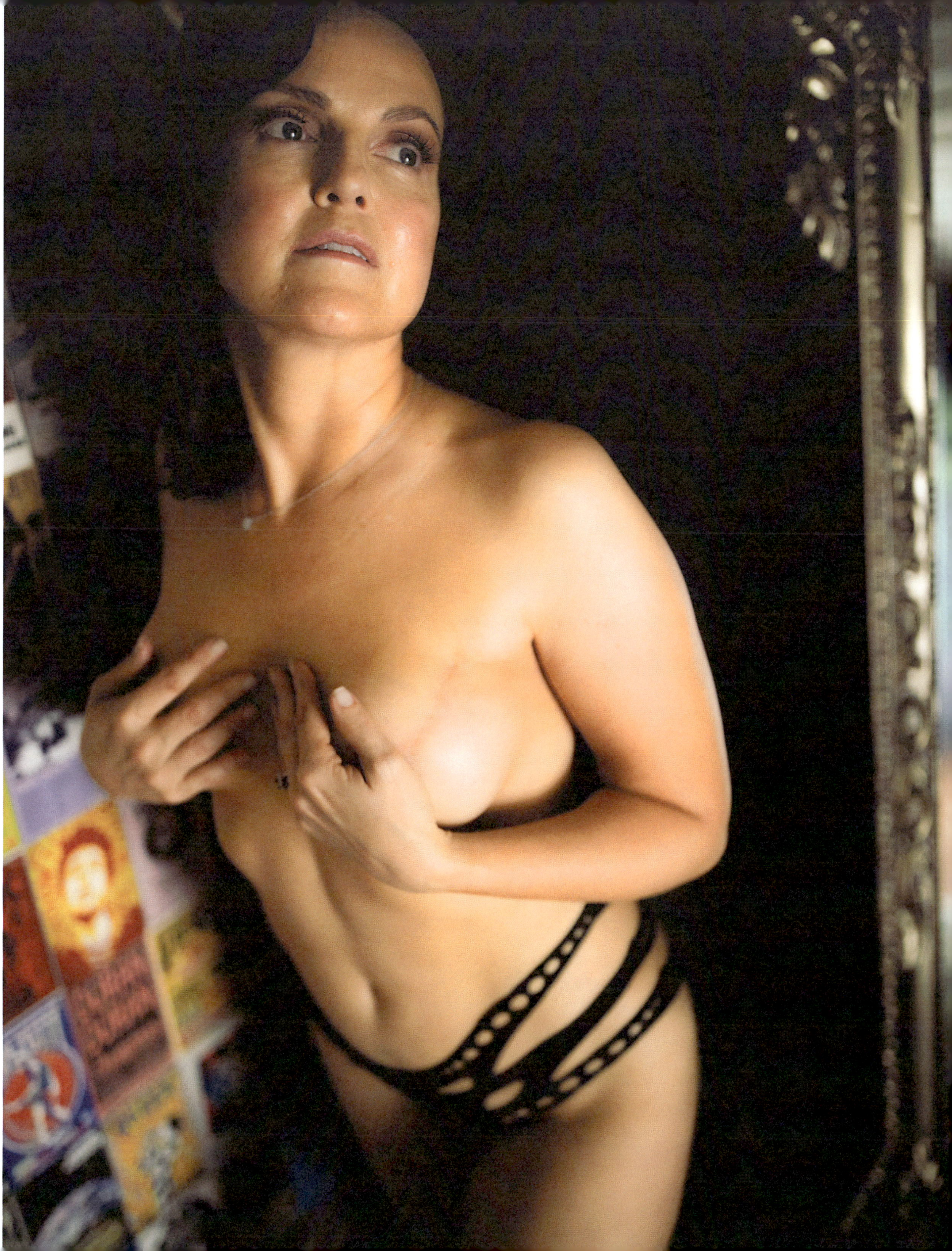

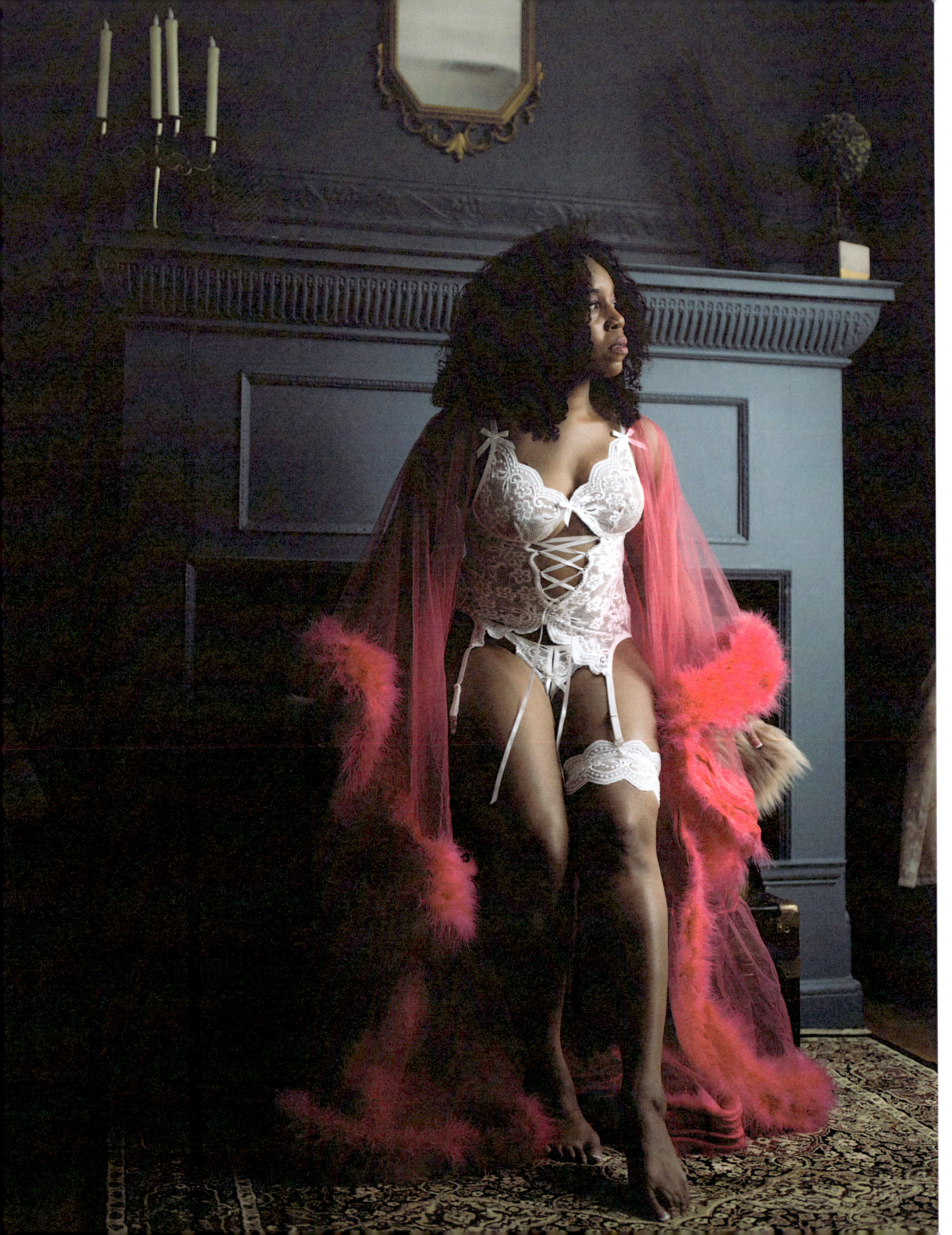

Diagnosis: Breast Cancer.
Age Diagnosed: 26 and 31
Treatments Received: Pill to shrink tumor, chemo, radiation, chemo. Mastectomy left side.
Age at time of photographs: 48
Stage at time of photographs: Survivor 17 years
Region: Bronx, NY
Social Media: @enhancebynature_

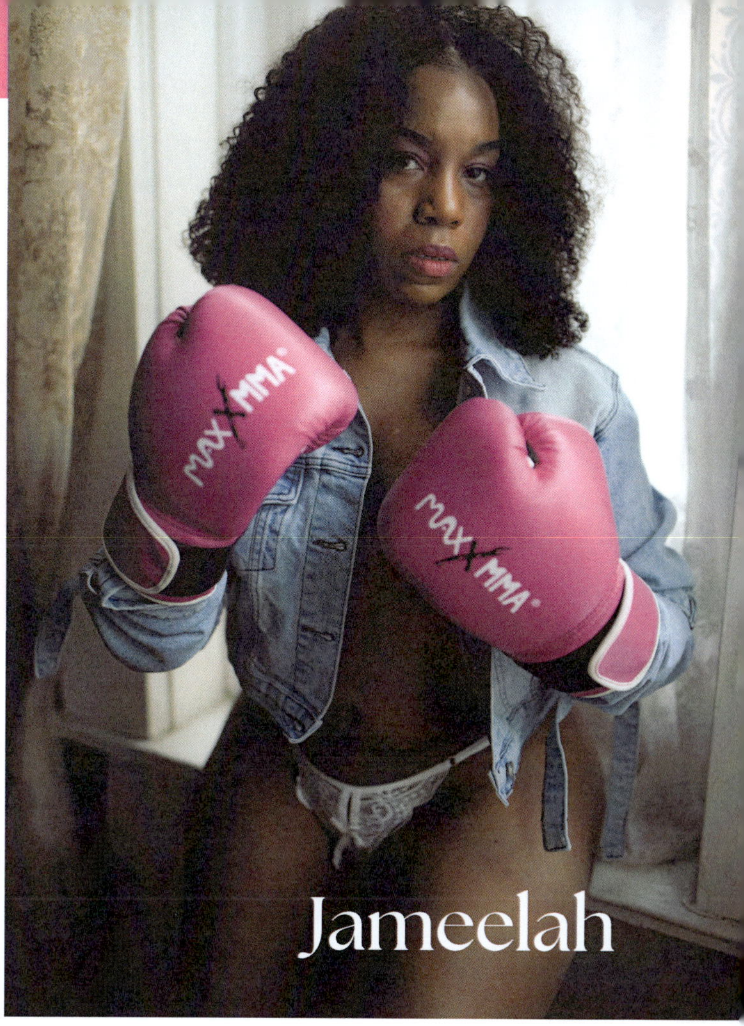

Jameelah

I'm proud to be a native of the Bronx, New York.

I graduated from the Fashion Institute of Technology, and I'm a mother to three incredible young men.

A transformative moment in my life occurred when I faced my first cancer diagnosis and completed my first round of chemotherapy.

The challenges I faced with my skin led me to realize the importance of taking control over what my family and I put on and in our bodies, divinely orchestrating my purpose.

For years, I started crafting skincare products for myself and my family. This led me to start my own skin care company: Enhanced By Nature.

After being diagnosed with breast cancer again five years later, my passion for interior design was reignited, a field I had long dreamed of pursuing. My mission was to design beautiful spaces that uplift our mental and emotional well-being as we return home from navigating our daily work lives.

A word of advice I would give to someone is: "You got this."

You have more support than you think, so utilize it. What you don't have, God will send your way.

A positive mindset can help you get through all the hard days.
Enjoy yourself, even though it's easier said than done. It's okay to let it out—cry, purge, write in a journal, release your feelings.

Your body will restore and heal itself as long as you rest, relax, pause, breathe, and learn to say things like, "I would love to, but I can't right now," or simply, "No."

Remember that saying no might take time to master, so give yourself grace.

My last words of wisdom, based on your experiences on the other side of this roadblock, are that this is a new chapter.

There is a new road and a new you ahead—don't be afraid to embrace it.

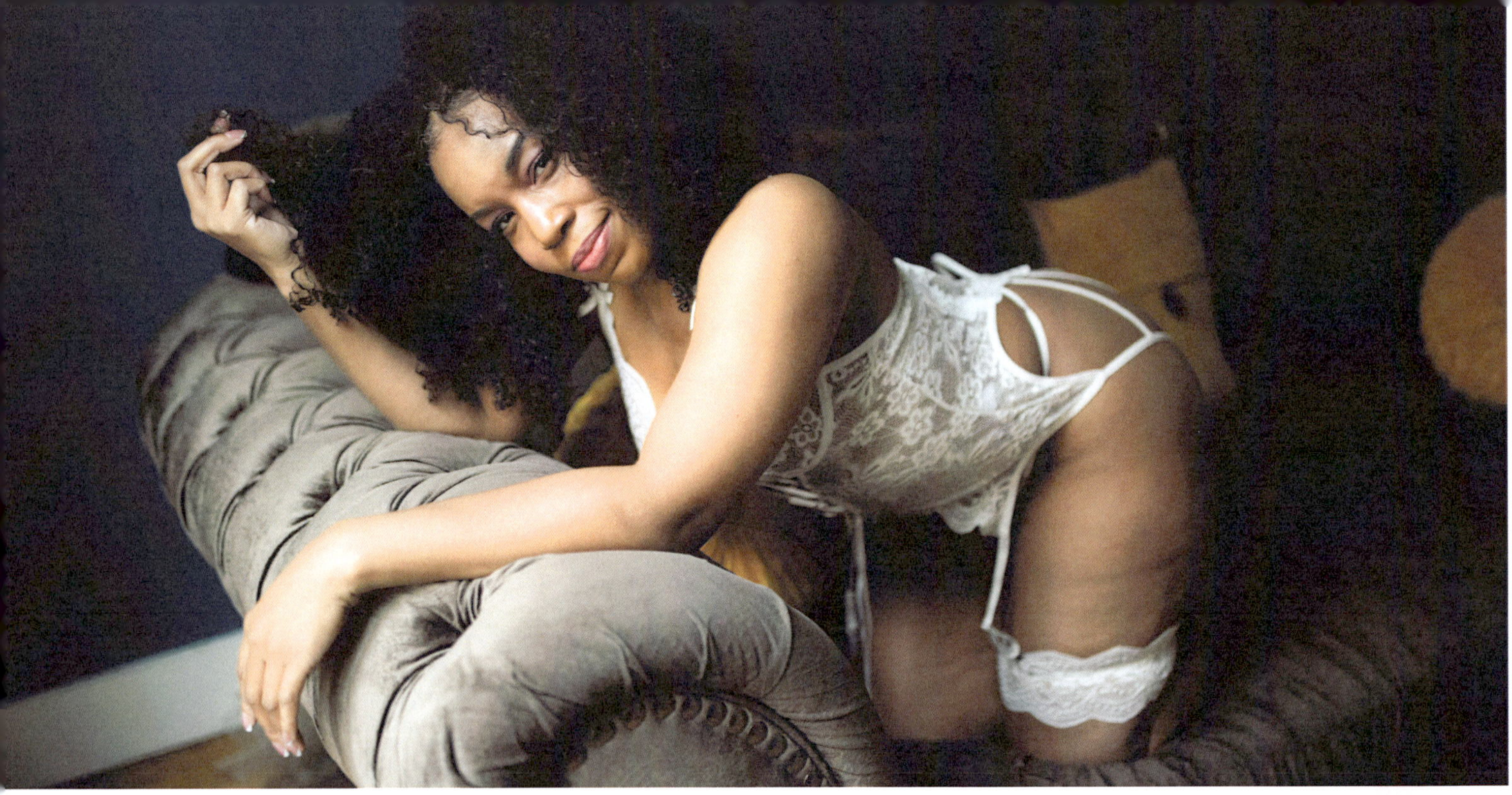

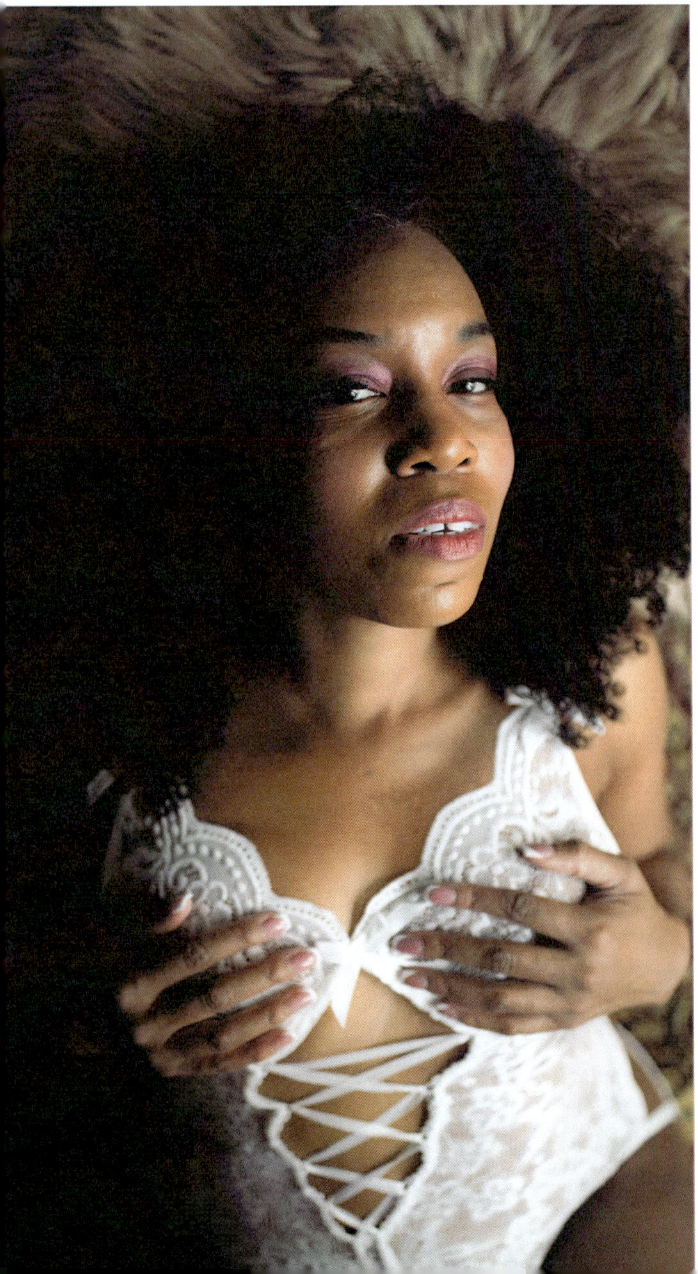

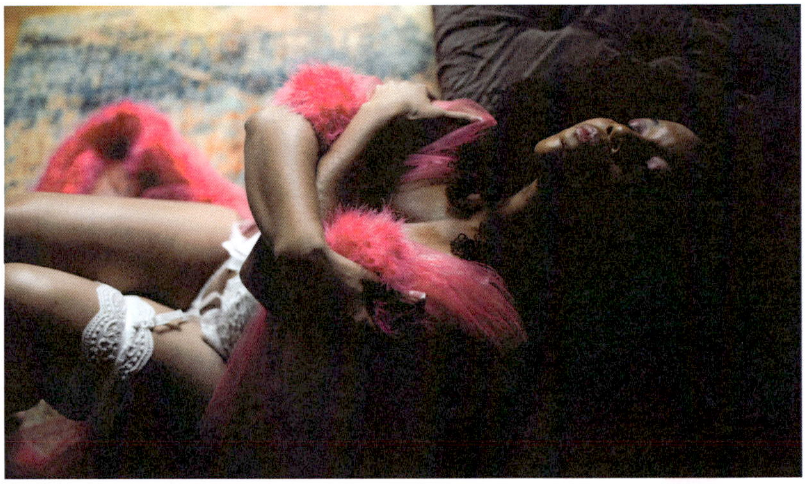

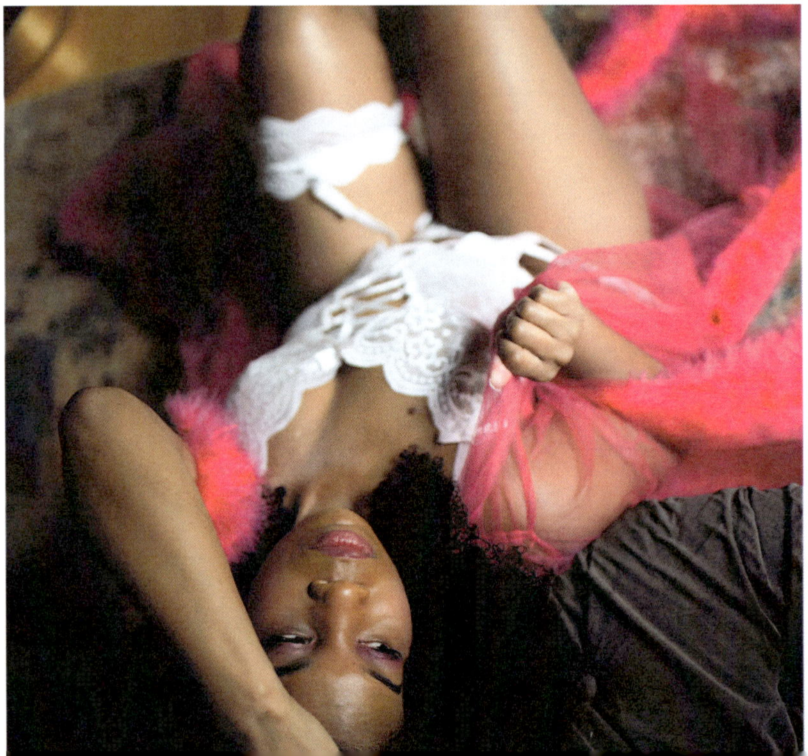

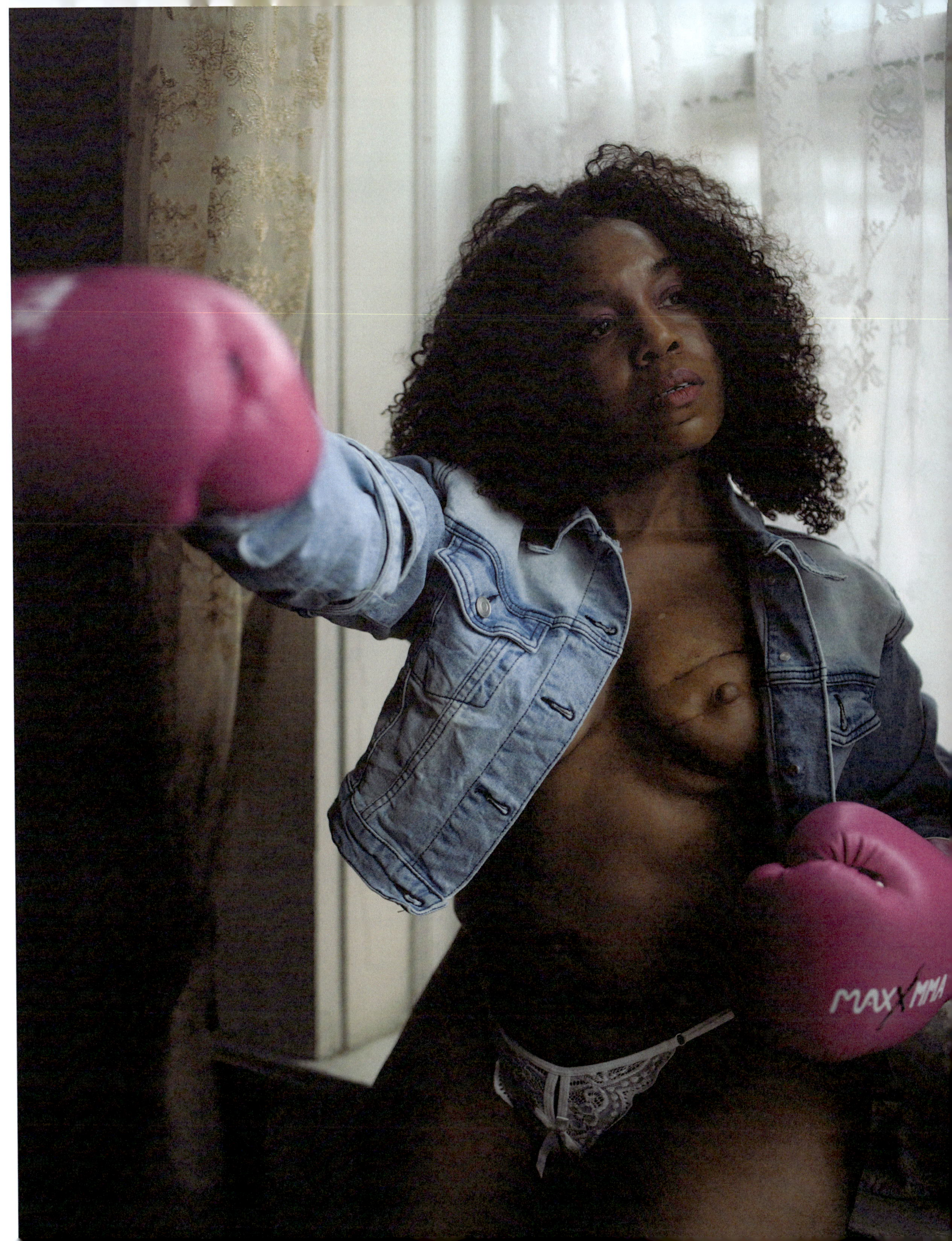
MAXxMMA

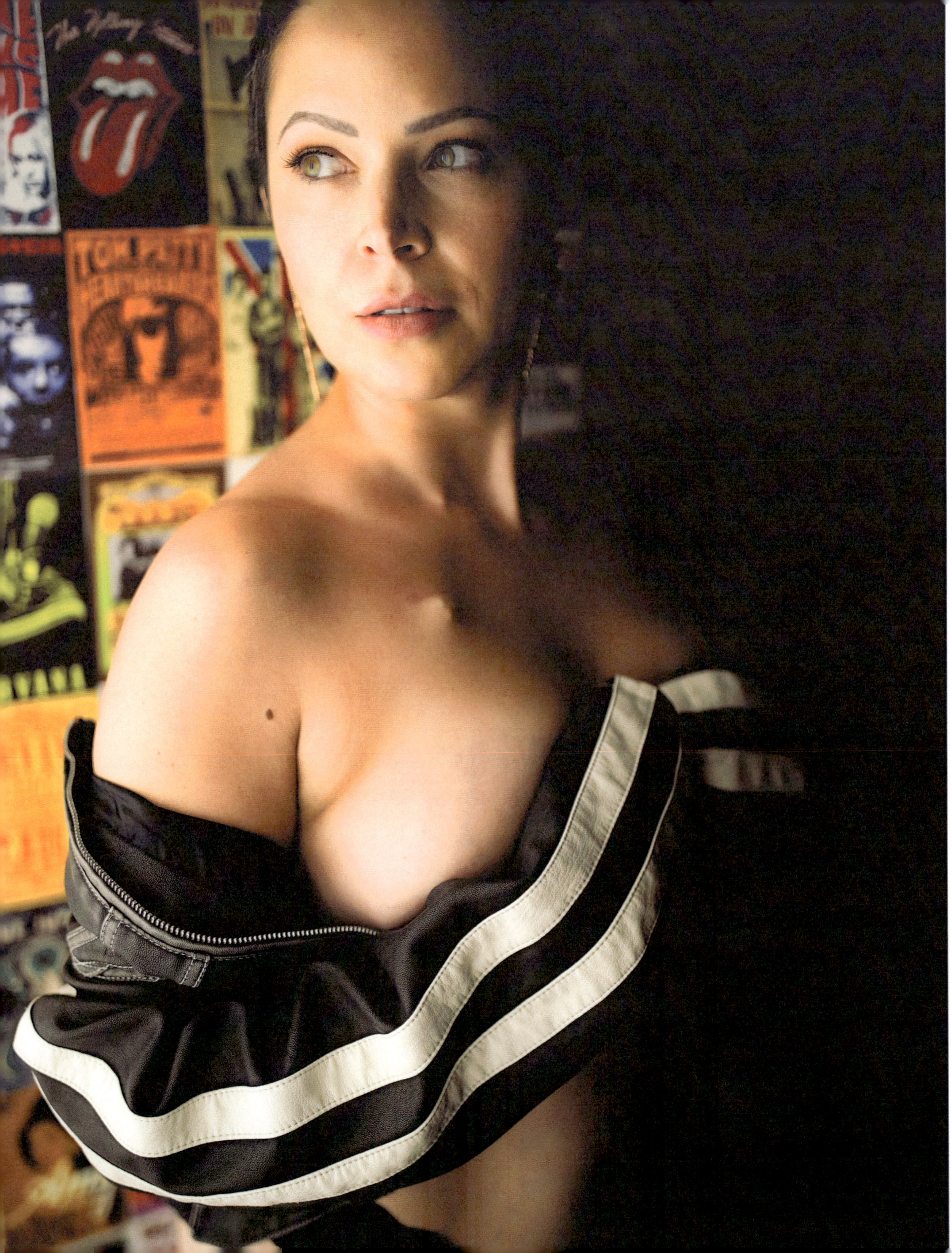

Kari

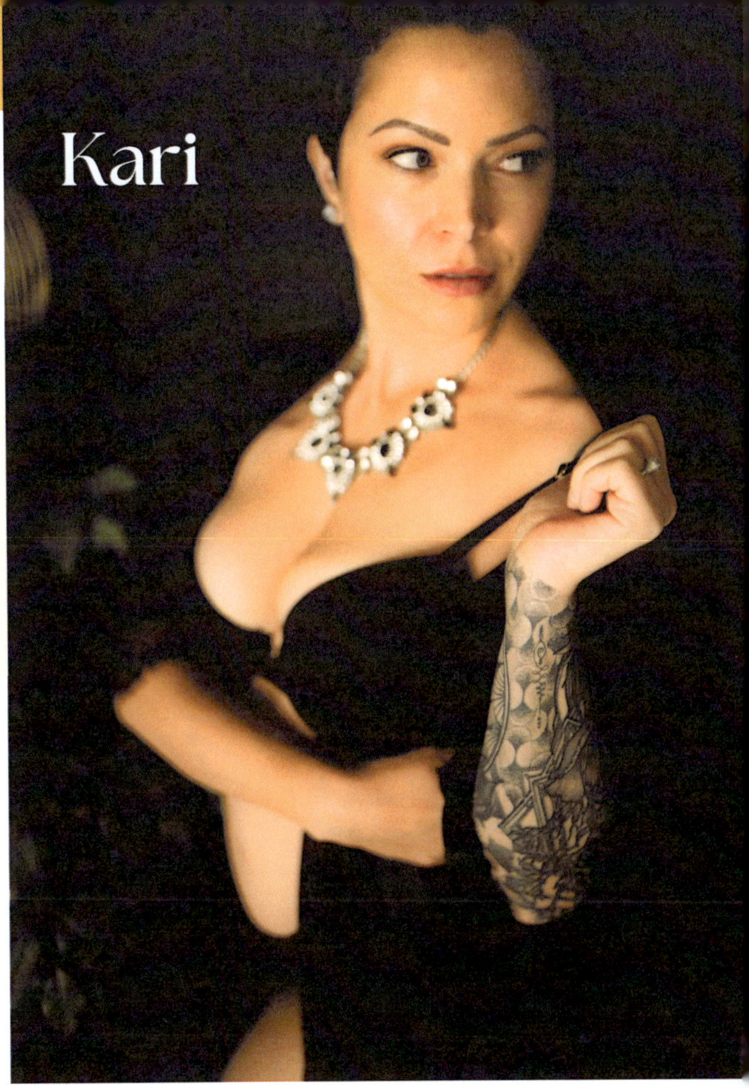

Diagnosis: De Novo Metastatic Invasive Ductal Carcinoma - Triple Positive.
Age Diagnosed: 37
Treatments Received: Chemotherapy, radiation to rib, double mastectomy with reconstruction, immunotherapy.
Age at time of photographs: 38
Stage at time of photographs: Stage 4
Region: Pacific Northwest

One of the first thoughts

that passed through my mind when I was first diagnosed with metastatic breast cancer was one of betrayal from my body.

How could my body have let this silent invader take hold and try to kill me?

Why wasn't it strong enough to detect and vanquish what felt like a trojan horse of an enemy?

I had many negative words in conjunction with my body and this illness. Weak, less than, imperfect, and so on.

After the initial few months, a lot of self reflection and therapy, the dynamic in my mind started to change.

I started looking at my body as a being who didn't need me talking about its flaws but treating it with love and gentleness.

I started recognizing how strong my body truly was for carrying me through life before cancer. My body holds so many stories of my life - both good and challenging.

My body had grown and given birth to my two amazing children.

Now, my body was holding strong through chemo and assisting in killing these silent invader cells.

The more I changed the conversation, the more me and my body felt like allies.

I no longer am afraid of my body betraying me, because I now understand we are partners.

I thank it for being so strong and for doing its best at keeping the cancer at bay.

I also now listen closer, when it asks me for rest or play.

Together we will face whatever the future may bring.

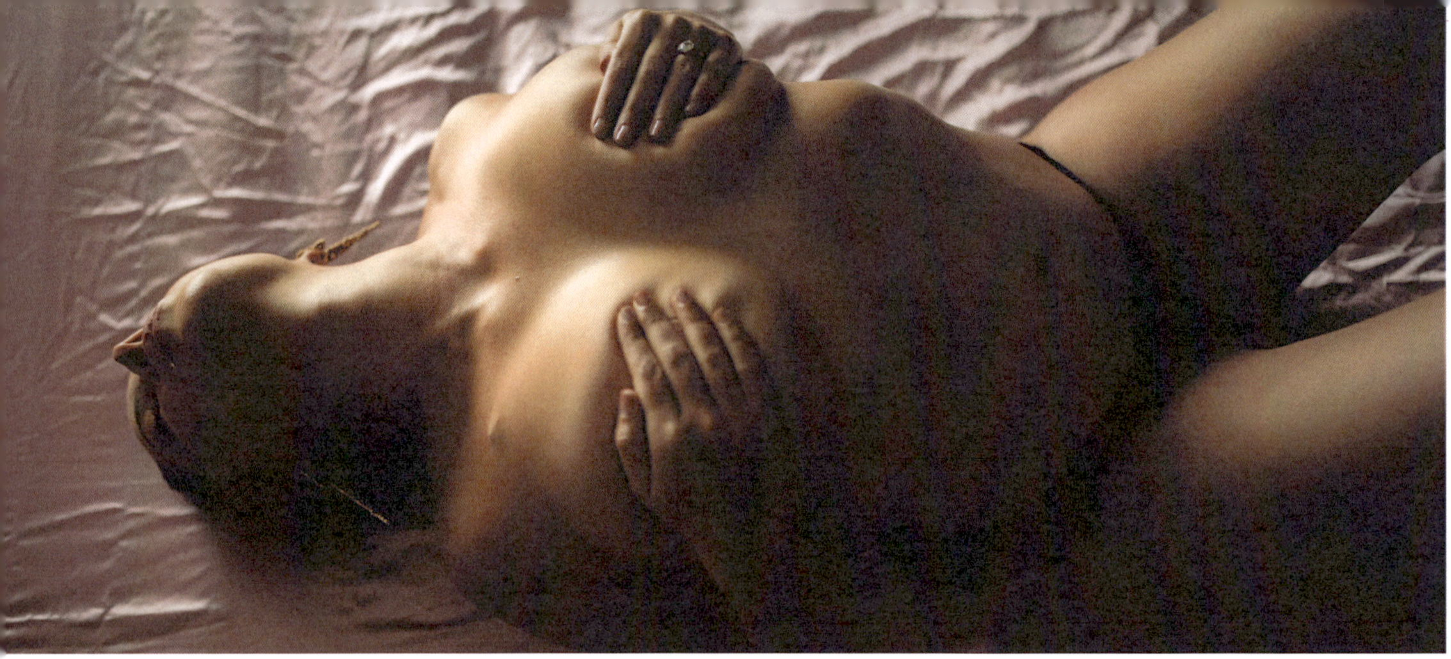

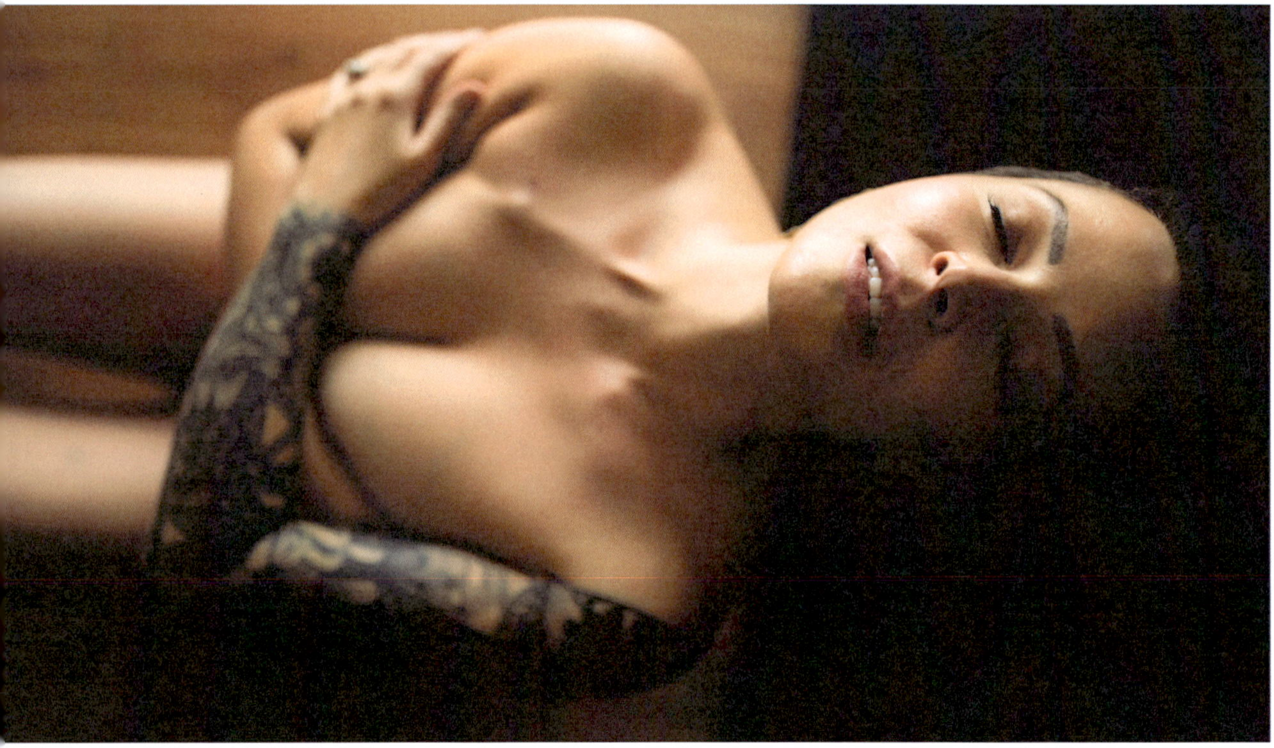

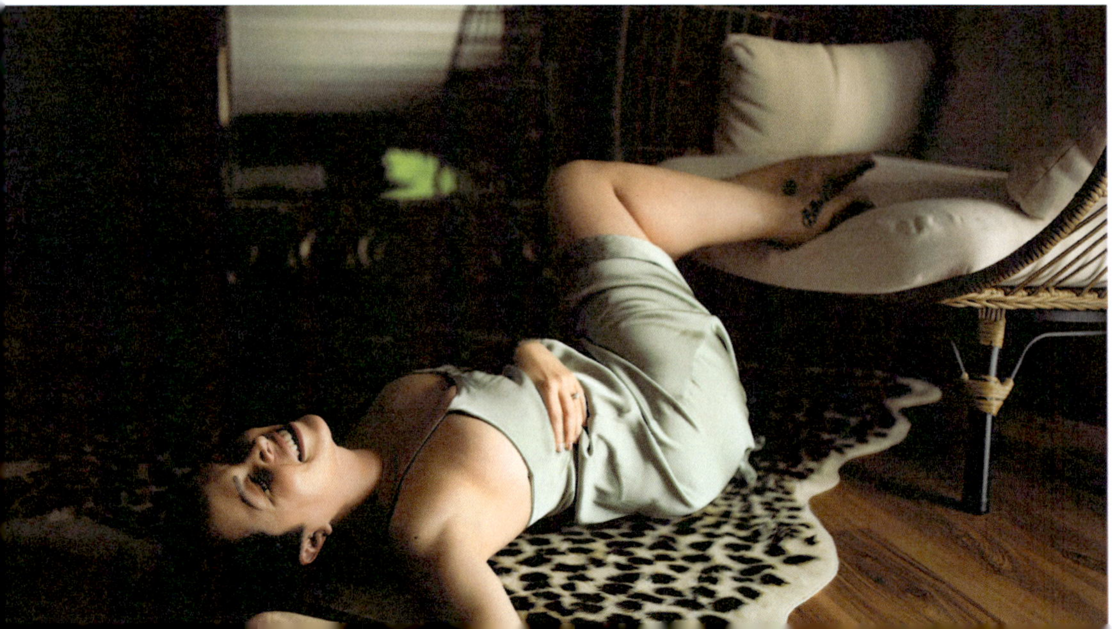

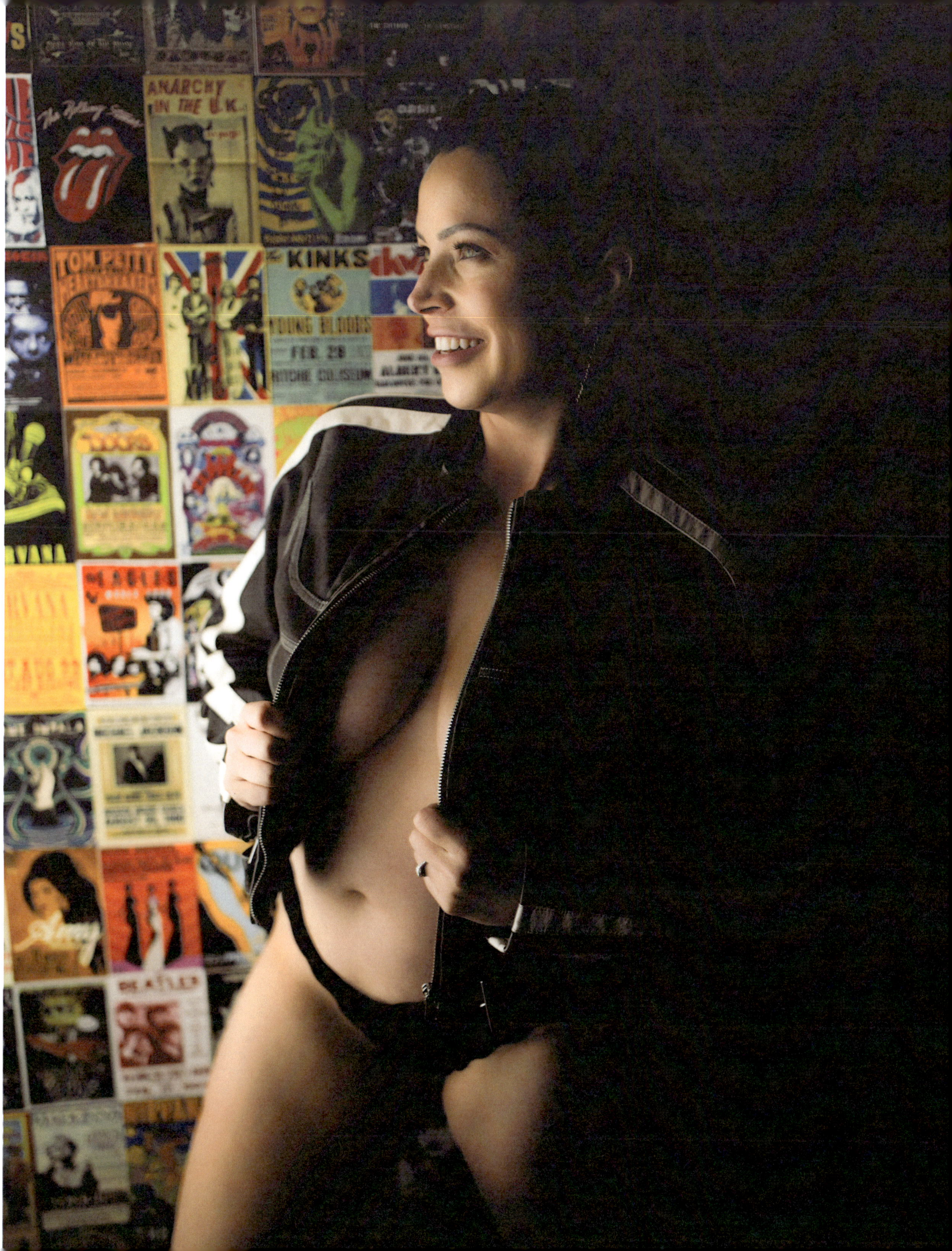
ANARCHY IN THE U.K.
TOM PETTY
THE KINKS
FEB. 28

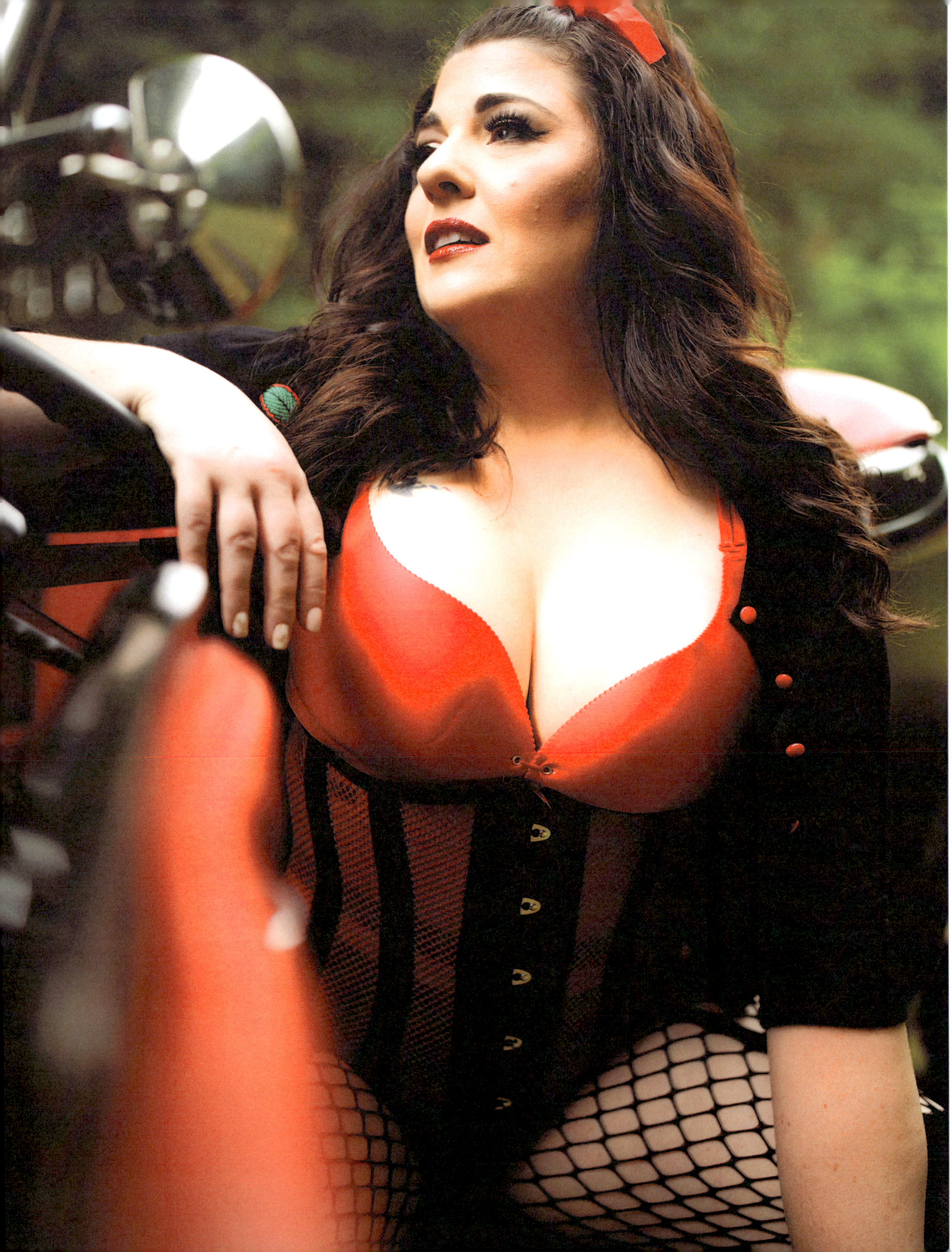

Katrina

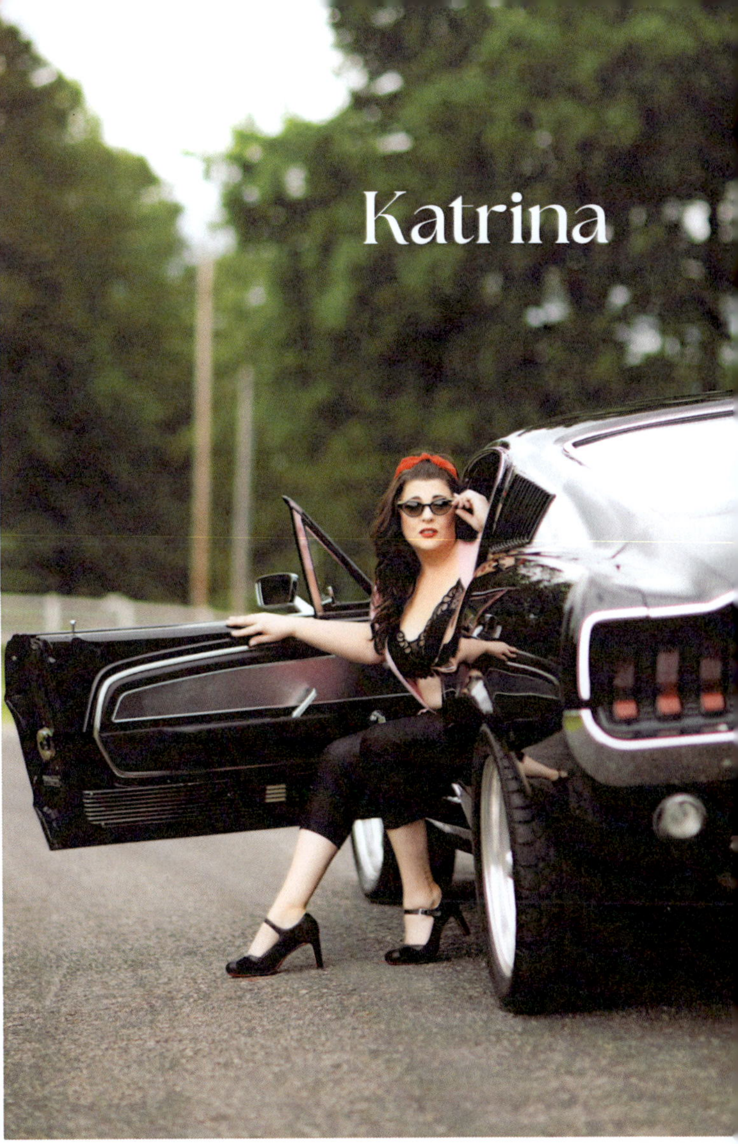

Diagnosis: Stage 3 Inflammatory Breast Cancer
Age Diagnosed: 42
Treatments Received: Chemotherapy and immunotherapy.
Age at time of photographs: 45
Stage at time of photographs: NED
Region: Western North Carolina
Social Media: @inflamed_cancer_ibc

This photo shoot was about capturing who I am and cars are a big part of my life. I grew up around them.

Auto shows on summer weekends were a must so this definitely shows who I am. Of course, this was also about confidence as a breast cancer survivor.

I have way more confidence now than I did before.

I take risks, I have fun, I meet new people, I don't care what people think, and I don't miss opportunities to show the world there is life after cancer.

It's a life worth living and if I can inspire one person, it's worth it.

As a breast cancer survivor, I went through so many physical and emotional changes.

As a breast cancer survivor, I went through so many physical and emotional changes.

Breast Cancer tore me down, but I've come back stronger than before.

I feel great inside and out.

I still can't believe this is me.

Life is beautiful, even when it's raining.

I was so happy the day I got this tattoo.
I finally had one small piece of control over something cancer had done to my body.

I wanted something to cover my chemo port scar.

I chose music notes because music got me through chemo.

I discovered so much music along the way that I created my own soundtrack for recovery and for life beyond cancer.

And the kitty is for my cat who always jumped on my port, made me scream in pain, but laid on top of it to comfort me when I was sick in bed from treatment.

I just hope that anyone going through cancer, in active treatment or on the other side of it can find their survivor voice and identity.

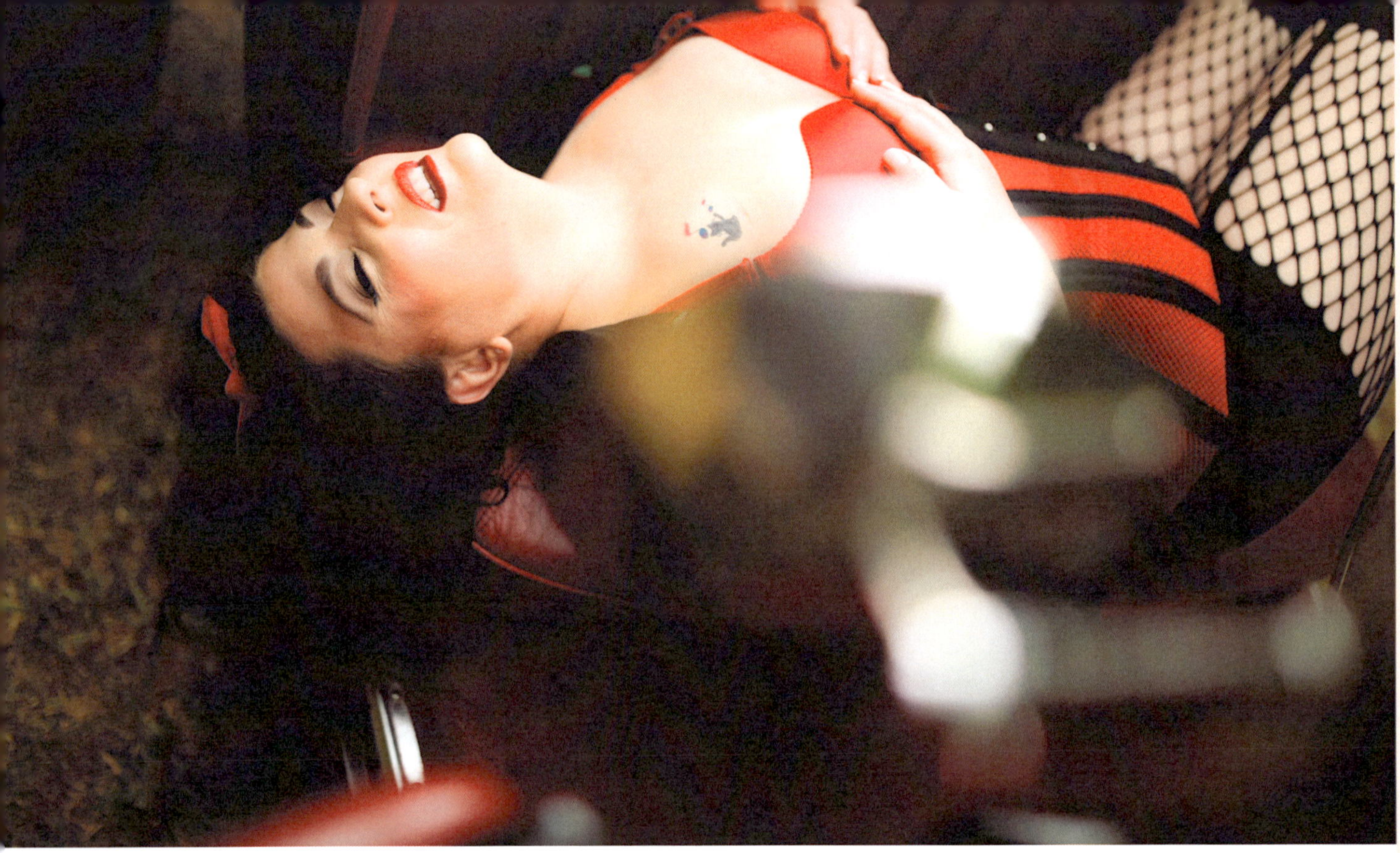

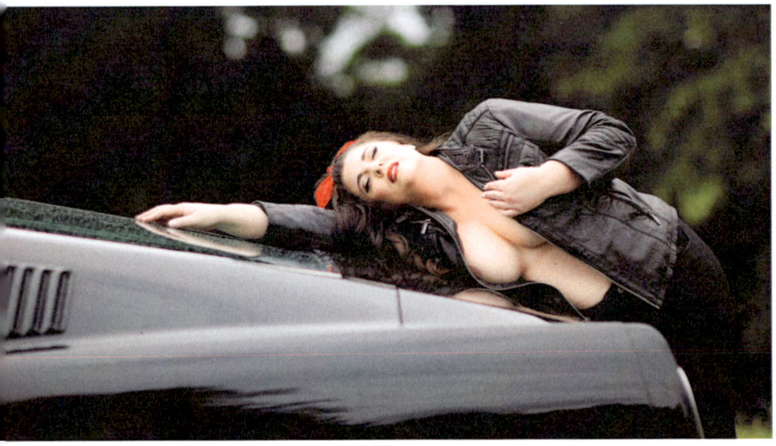

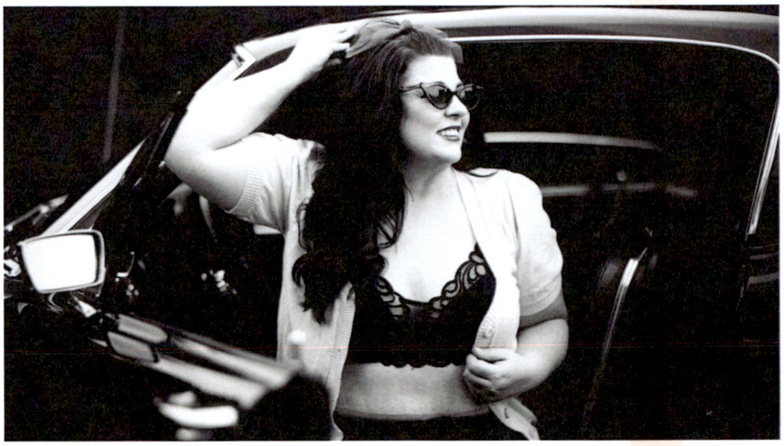

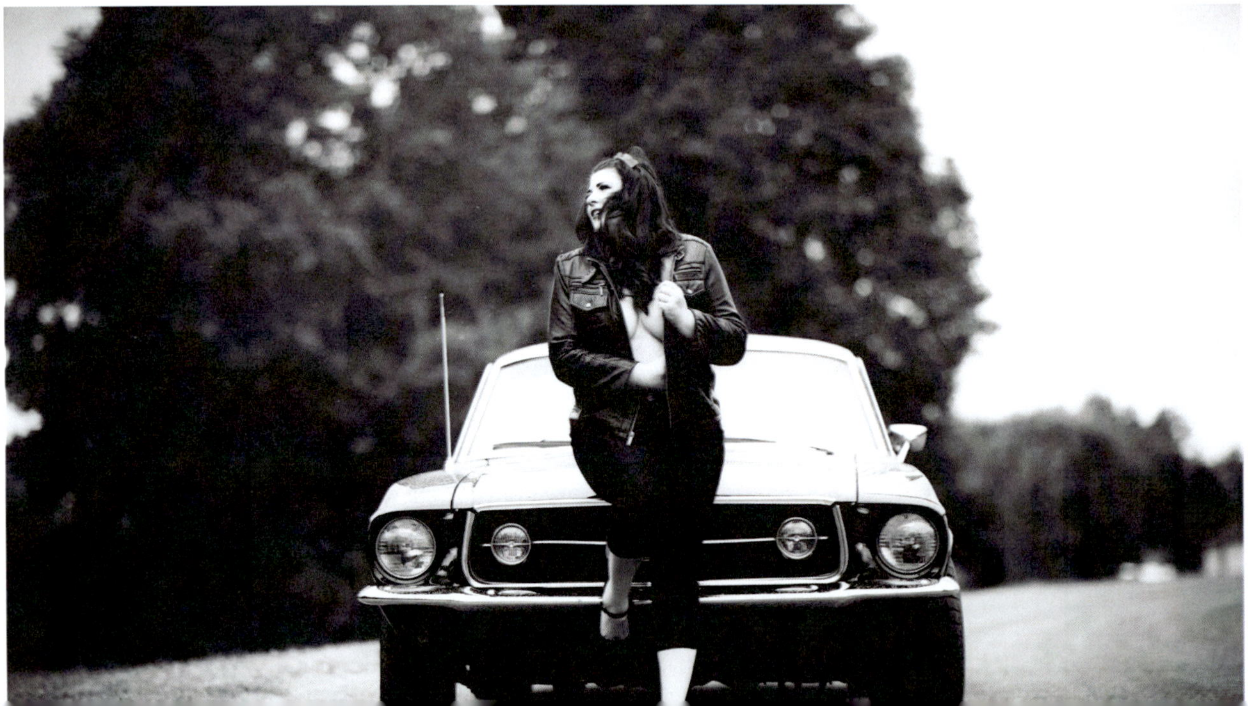

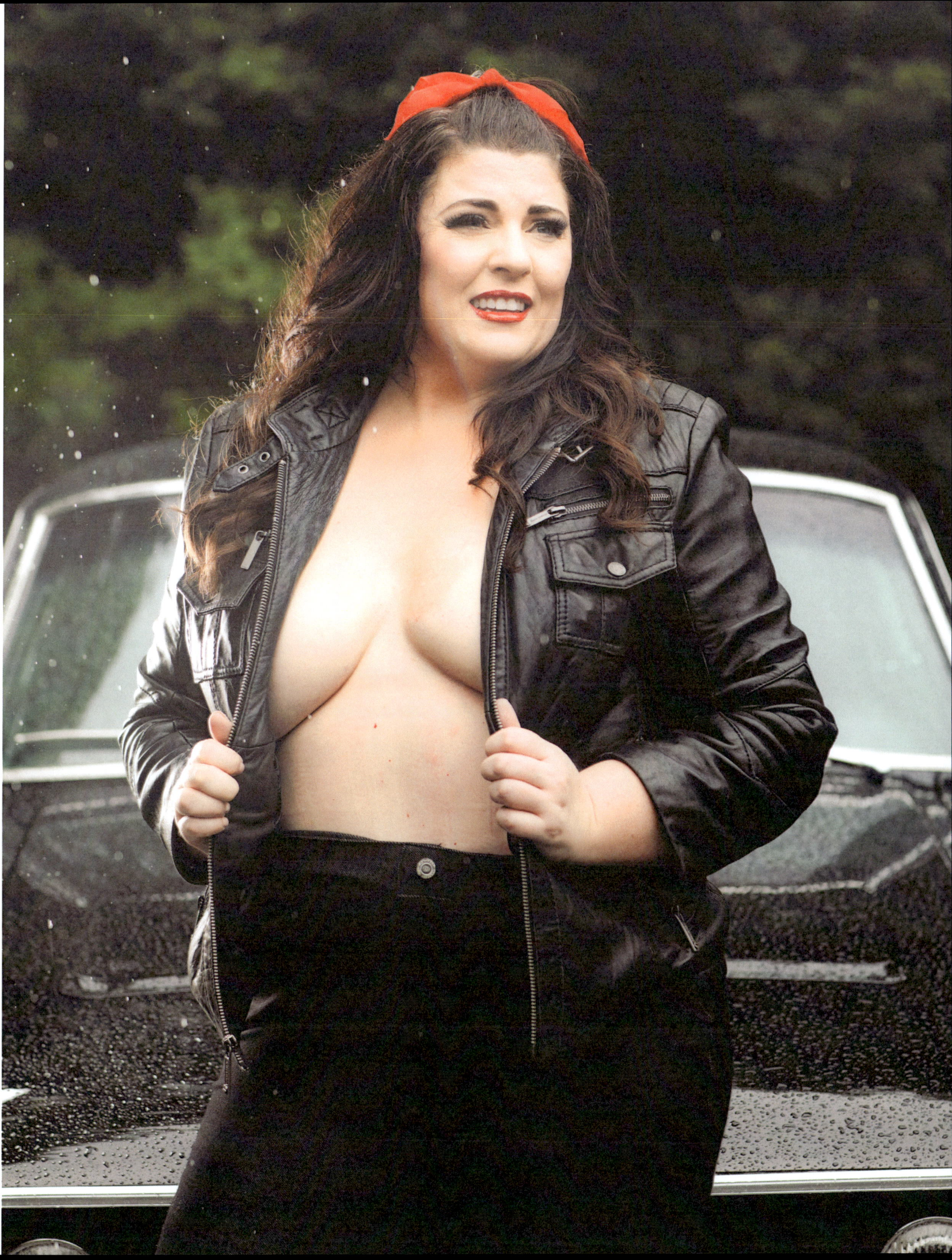

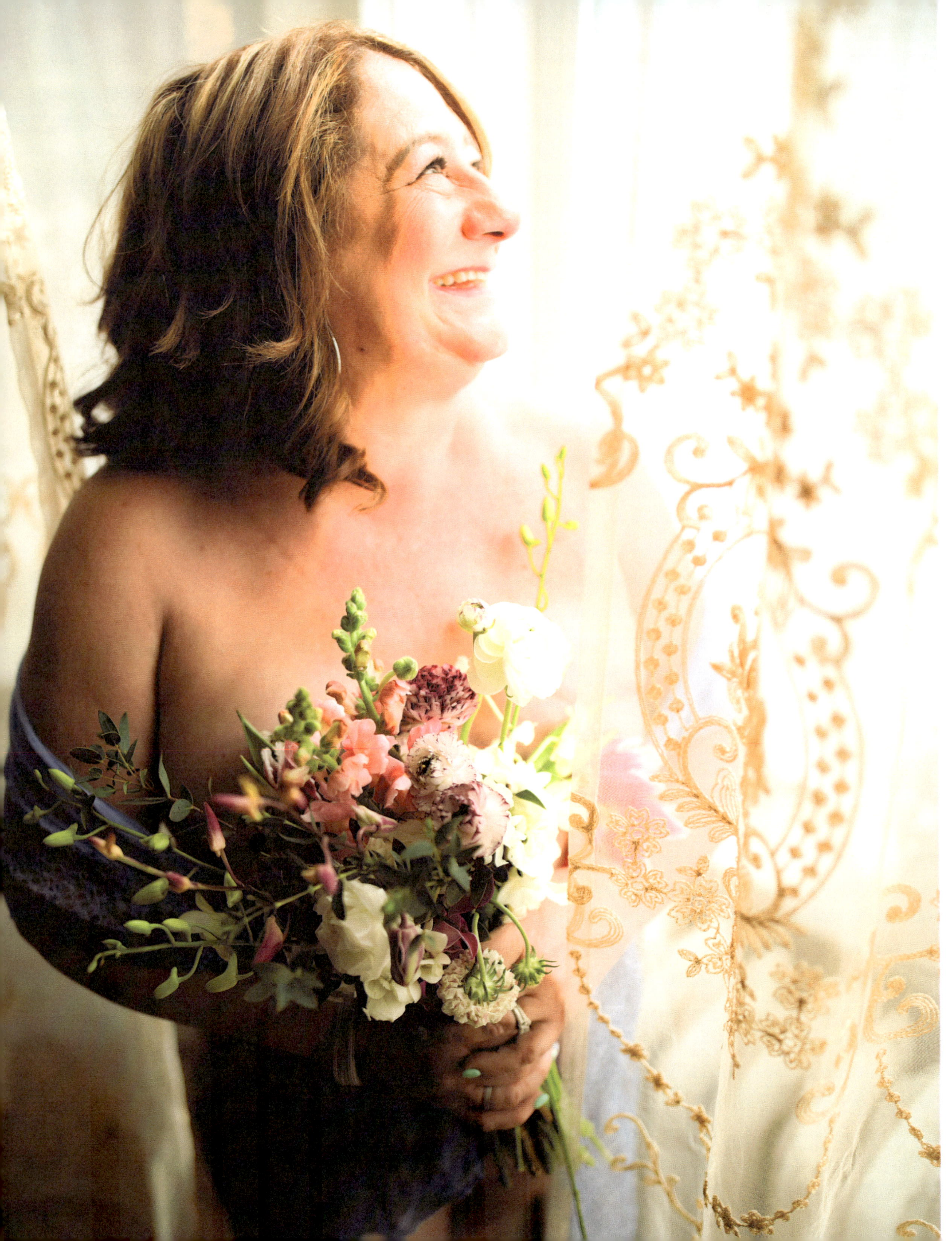

Diagnosis: *Stage 3 Breast Cancer.*
Age Diagnosed: *31*
Treatments Received: *8 rounds of chemotherapy, 4 rounds of oral chemo.*
Age at time of photographs: *41*
Stage at time of photographs: *Remission*
Region: *Northeast*

My breast cancer journey wasn't an easy one—although who's is?

My son was 10 months old when I was diagnosed. I remember the call like it was yesterday.

I remember feeling like I failed him, because my daughter nursed for 16 months, and now here I was weaning him at 10 months old.

I slept on the couch while my husband tried to bottle feed him, his cries so sad and pitiful. I pumped and pumped and pumped. I wanted to have as much as I could stored up for him before I started eight rounds of aggressive chemotherapy.

I gave very little thought to my needs or feelings throughout my entire journey. there just didn't seem to be time for that.

Everyday I was getting up, looking in the mirror and brushing off the thoughts I had. I thought I was unhappy with how I looked before? Nothing prepared me for how I was going to look after surgery. 4 drains, no hair, and a body that looked like a sewn up rag doll.

I started to realize somewhere deep down, past the scars (battle wounds), past the wig covering mousey brown hair, there was someone there I hadn't seen in quite some time. There was the person there, who realized she didn't fight to live, to live unhappy.

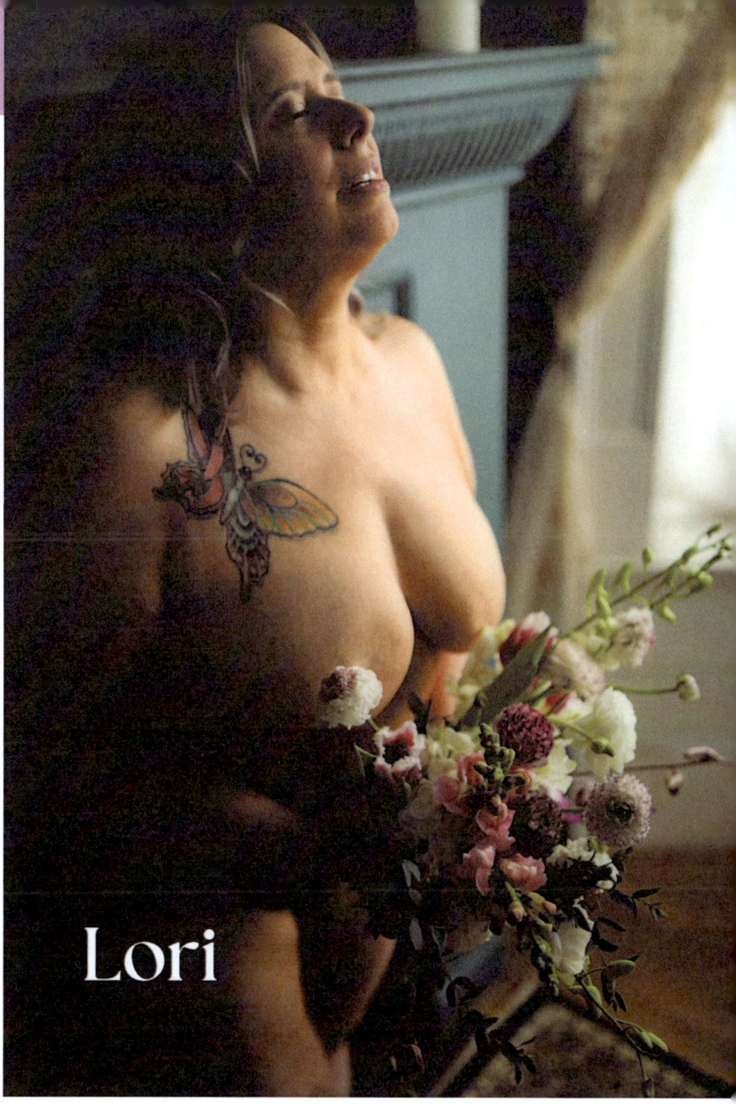

Lori

My life changed dramatically, but as it changed around me, I changed too. I realized that cancer wasn't bad if I learned something good from it.

I found a spark and fight in me I didn't know I had.

Through it all I started to see myself as beautiful, not for how I looked in the mirror, but for how I looked to my daughter and son, who looked at me the same as they always had.

As their mama.

As beautiful, strong, and the person they loved more than anyone in the world.

The love and growth was what made me feel better about myself again, and one day, I looked in the mirror with my new husband standing behind me, and saw the beautiful woman he and everyone else saw all along...I just had to find her.

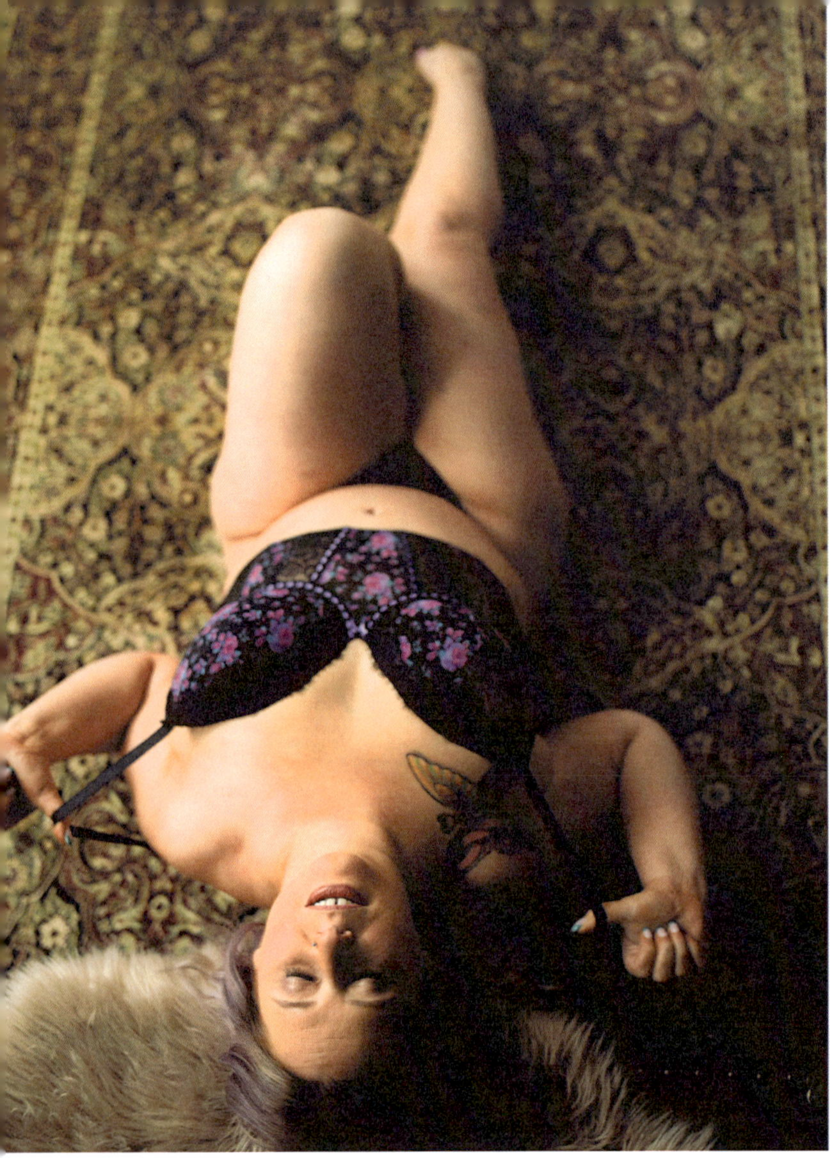

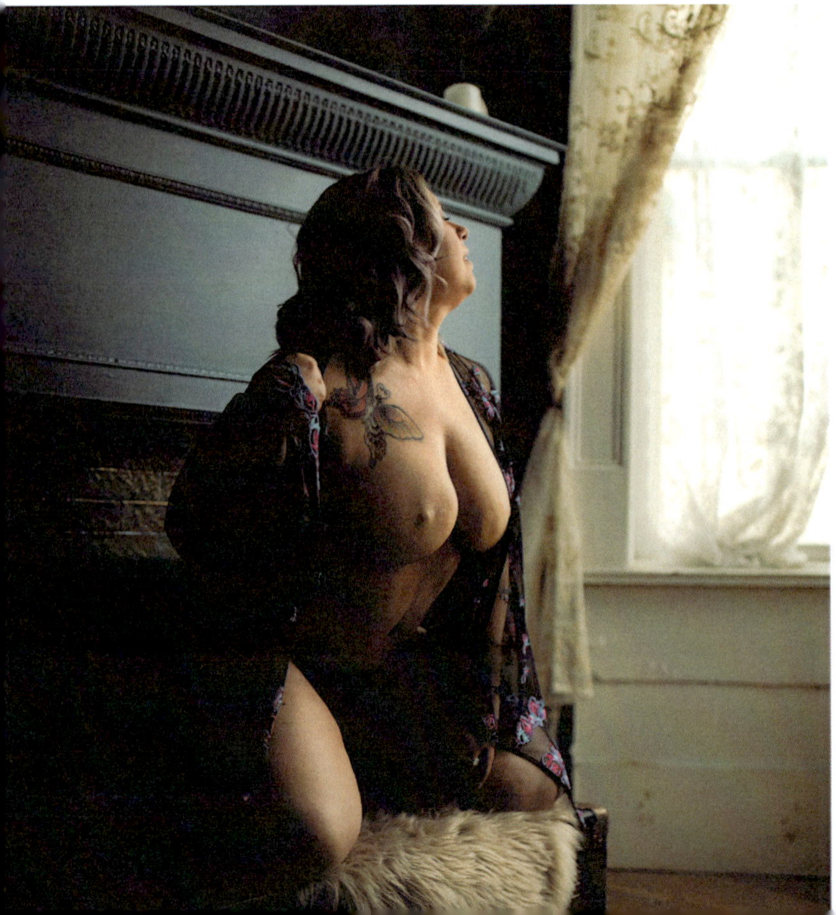

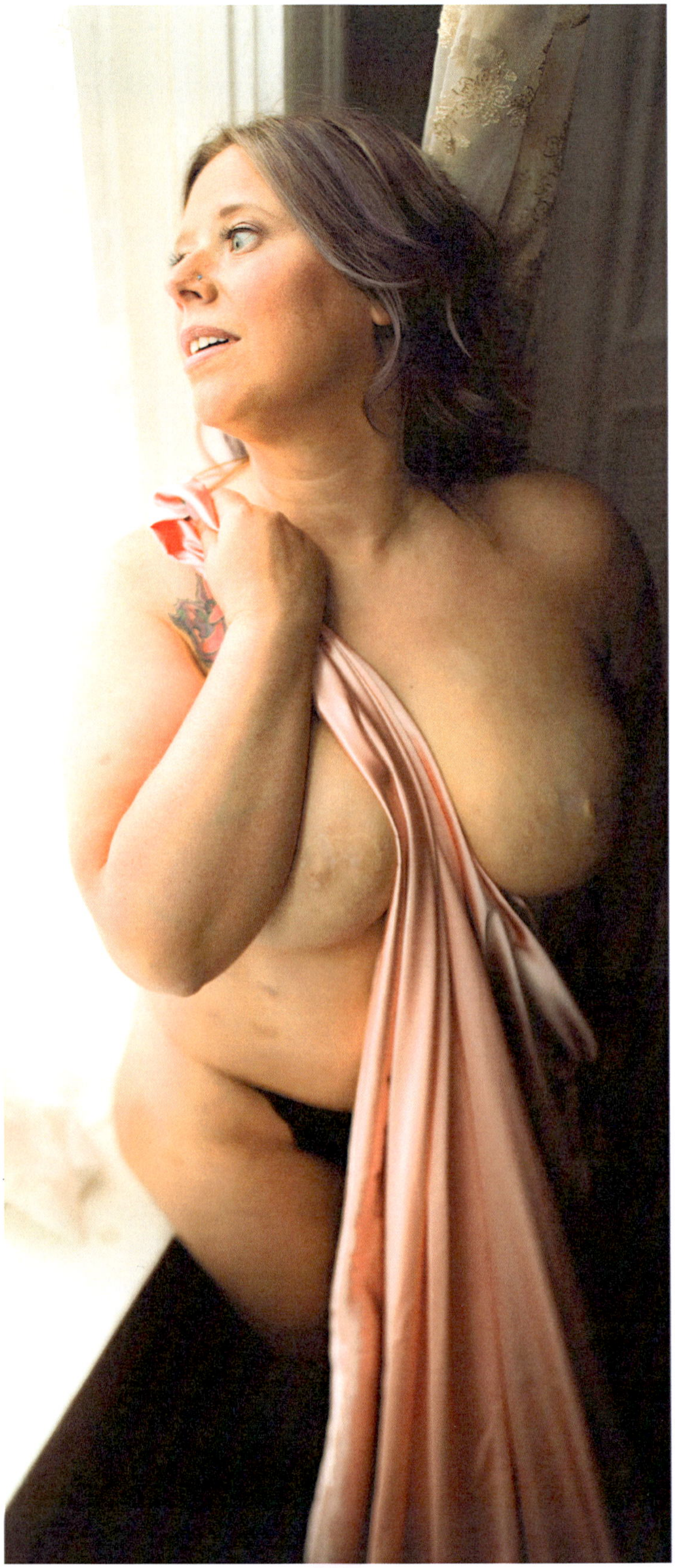

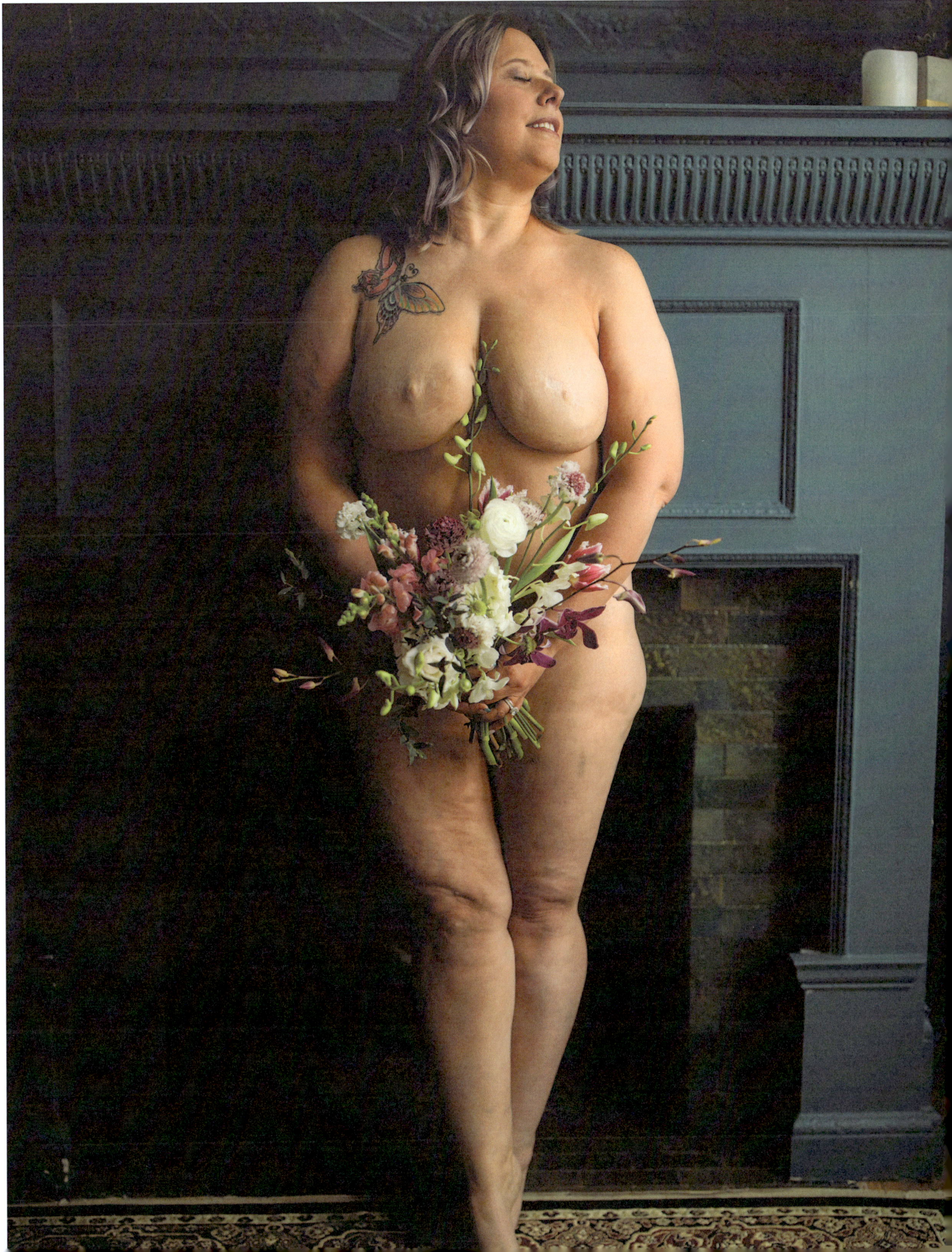

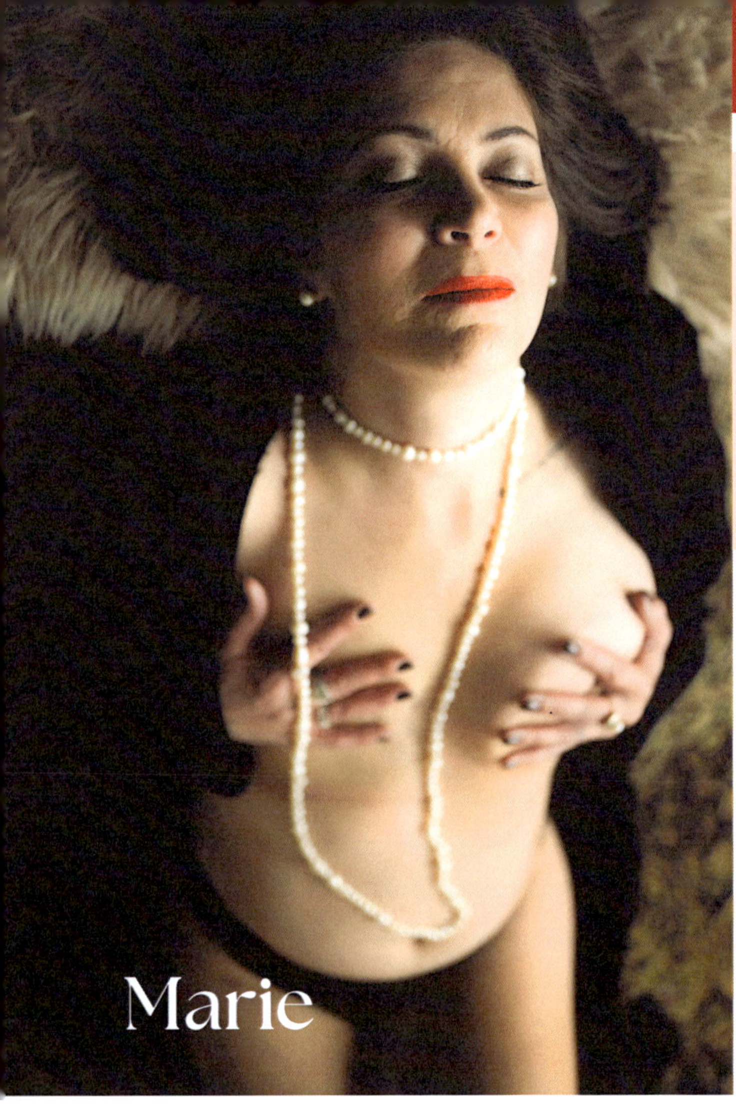

Marie

Diagnosis:	*Stage 3 Lobular Breast Cancer Estrogen Positive.*
Age Diagnosed:	*44*
Treatments Received:	*Mastectomy, Chemotherapy, Radiation, Lymph Node dissection and medications.*
Age at time of photographs:	*46*
Stage at time of photographs:	*Completed all active treatment aside from medication.*
Region:	*Canada*
Social Media:	*@Tittalkwithyourbreastie*

I am a passionate advocate, volunteer, blogger, mother, wife, and grandmother,

driven by a personal journey that began with my diagnosis of Lobular Breast Cancer at 44.

Having walked the path of both cancer survivor and caregiver, I've come to believe in the transformative power of connection.

Every conversation is an opportunity to inspire someone to take control of their health or offer support to a loved one.

Cancer may be a daunting adversary, but it has also given me a renewed sense of purpose. It has strengthened my resolve to leave behind a legacy of hope, resilience, and empowerment for generations to come.

Through my work, I strive to make a meaningful impact, knowing that even the hardest battles can lead to a brighter, more purposeful life.

The mental and emotional toll of cancer was something I could never have fully prepared for.

After my mastectomy, I struggled with my identity and femininity. Yet, amid the pain and uncertainty, I found beauty in my journey.

Unexpected experiences, like participating in the Breast Cancer Confidence Project with The Photography Experience, allowed me to see myself through a new lens.

I learned to embrace the beauty of my scars and realized that every challenge only deepened my strength and grace.

Cancer, though it takes much from you, also gives back in surprising ways. It's an unwelcome guest that overstays its welcome but leaves you with a profound new perspective on life.

Through this journey, I've learned what truly matters—what's worth my time, and who is deserving of it. Along the way, I've met extraordinary women whose compassion and support have filled my heart with gratitude and joy.

I'm proud to serve as the Custom Breast Form Ambassador for Amoena Canada. In making the decision not to pursue reconstruction, I want every woman to know that there are choices.

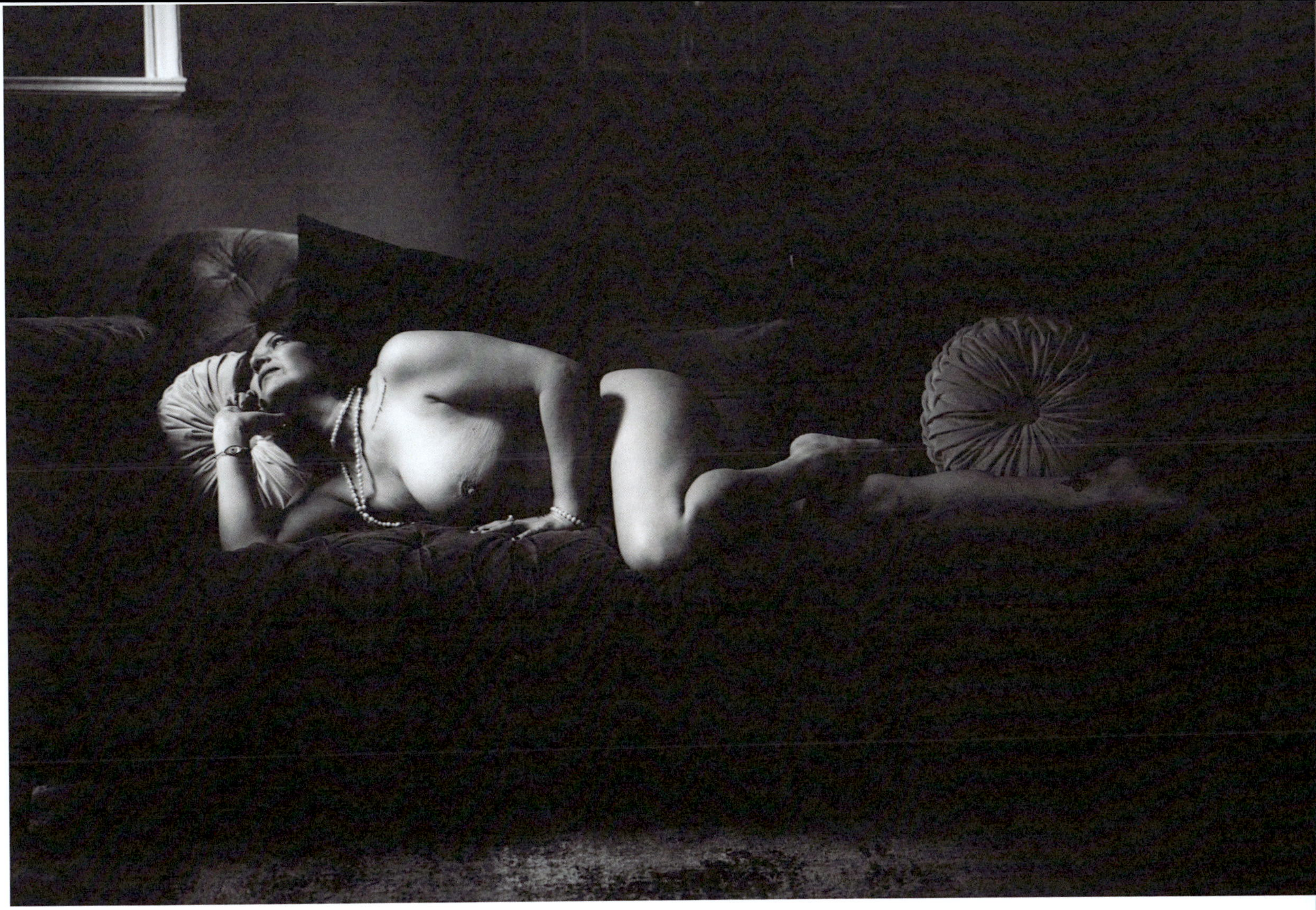

For me, undergoing another surgery felt daunting and risky, especially considering my history with open-heart surgeries as a child. Instead, having a custom breast form has been a true blessing — it's allowed me to feel whole again and continue thriving, embracing my new path with confidence.

It turns out that cancer doesn't just take you places physically—it transforms you in ways you never expected.

Reflecting on the past few years—through the highs, the lows, and the countless blessings I never saw coming—I am filled with gratitude.

Grateful to still be here, thankful for the fresh outlook on life, and incredibly appreciative of the beautiful friendships that have blossomed from this journey.

Sharing my story has taught me more about myself than I ever imagined.

These experiences have shown me that cancer, though it may take you on an unexpected path, can lead you to places of profound growth and connection.

Cancer may not have been the best life coach, but it certainly taught me some invaluable lessons. It taught me to make time, take time, and cherish every moment.

In a world that moves too quickly, I have learned that the most precious moments are the ones we are fully present for. It's in the love we give, the laughter we share, and the strength we find in one another.

These are the moments that shape us and remind us what truly matters.

Embrace it ! Be your own Breastie.

(#tittalkwithyourbreastie)

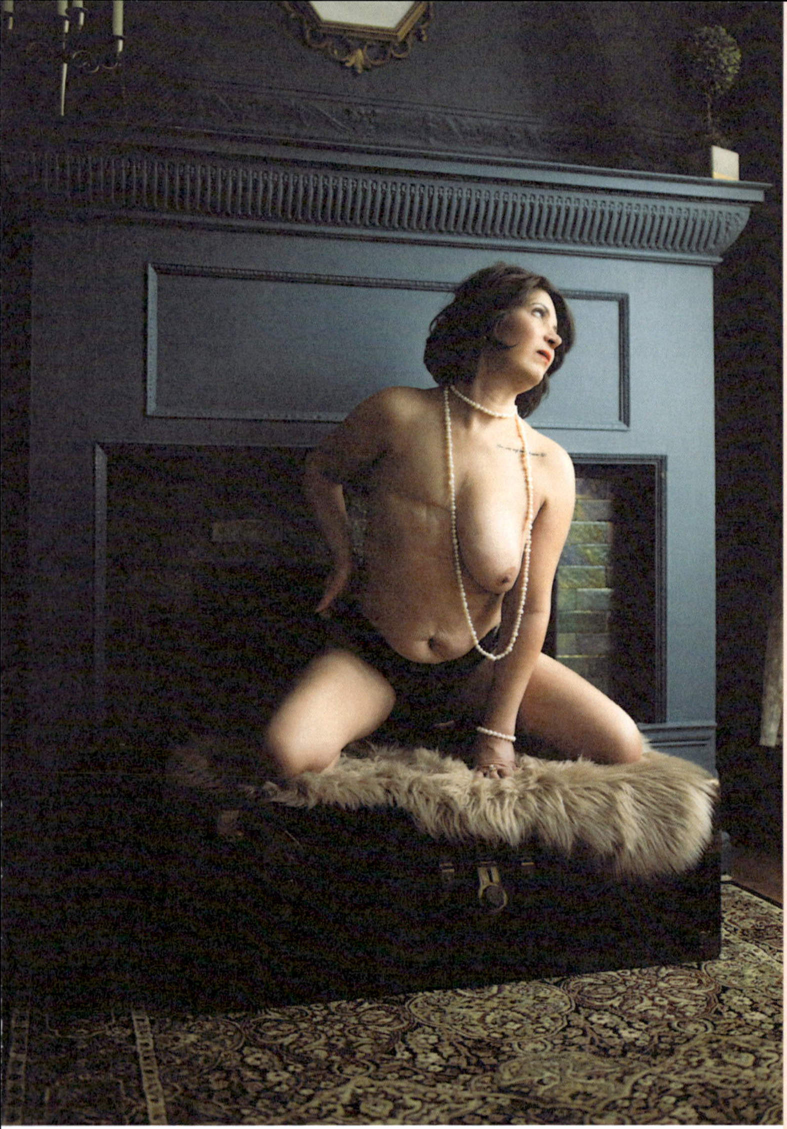
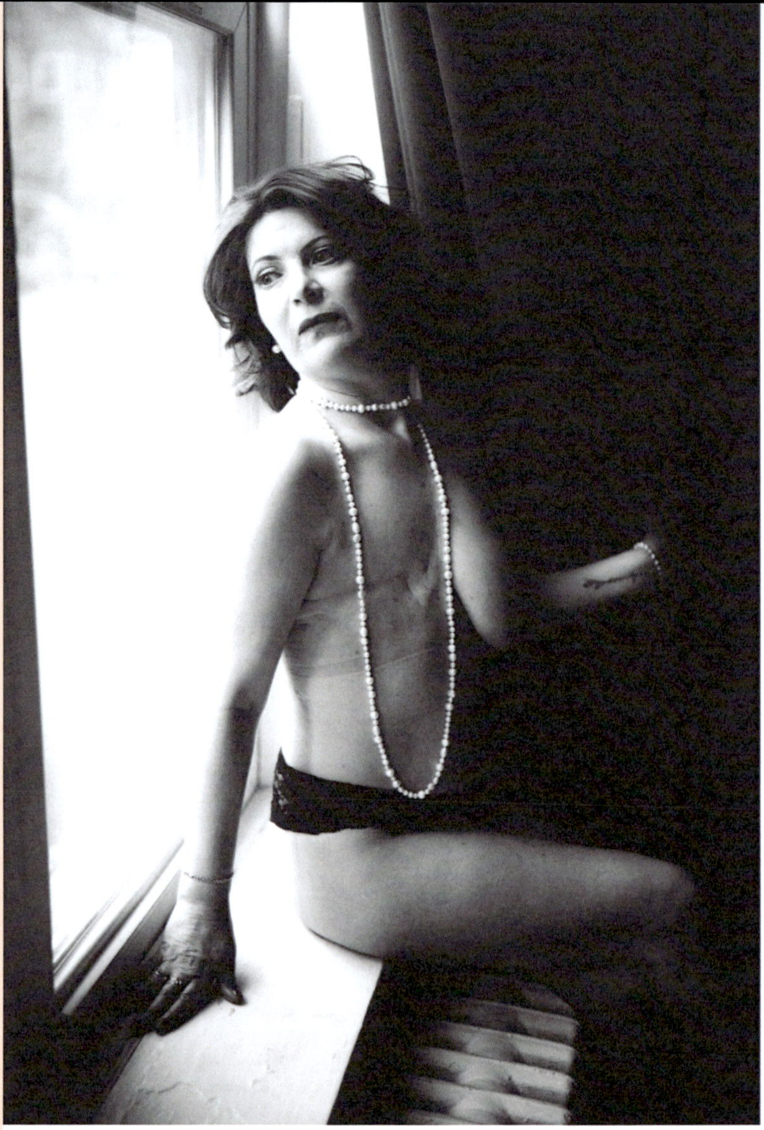
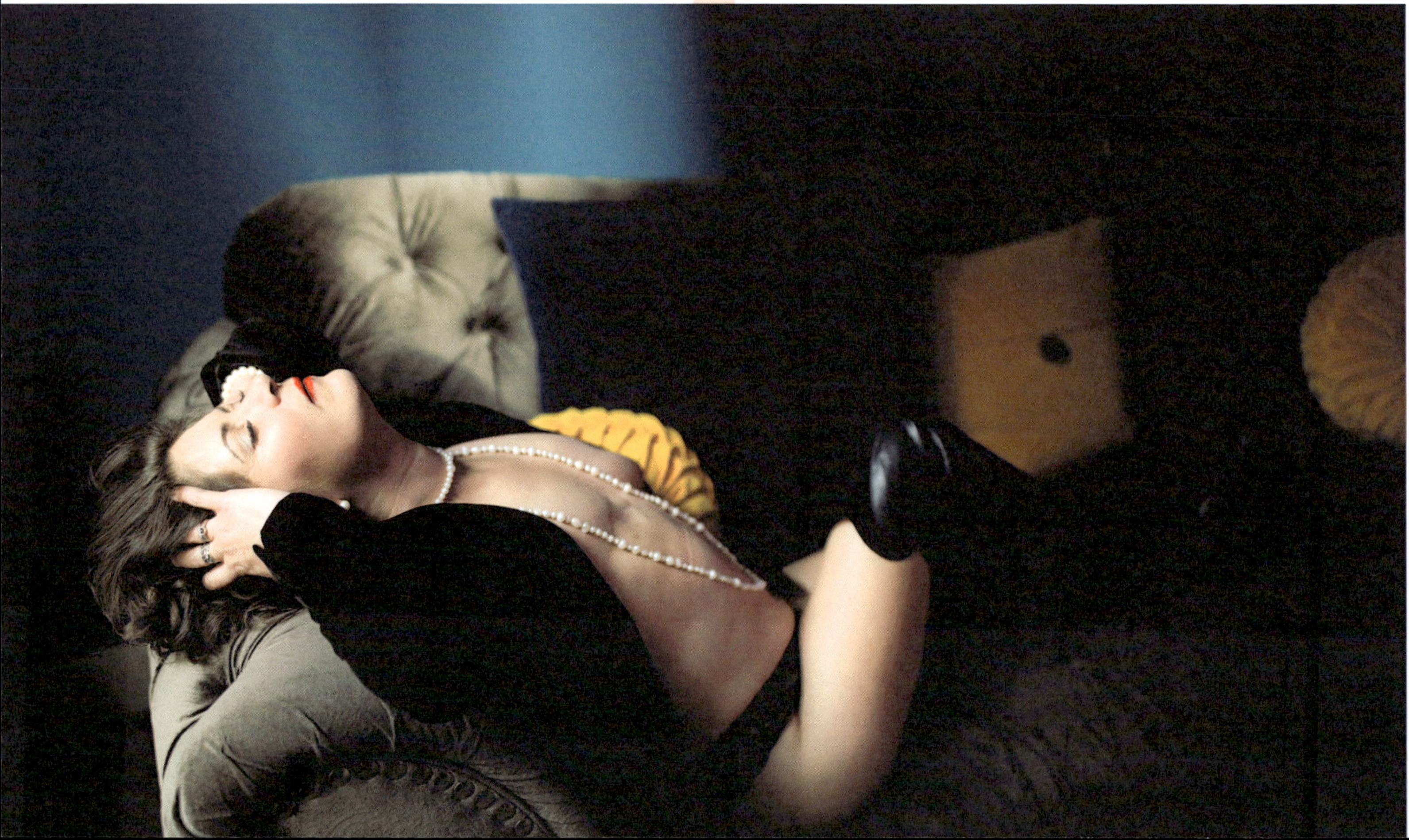

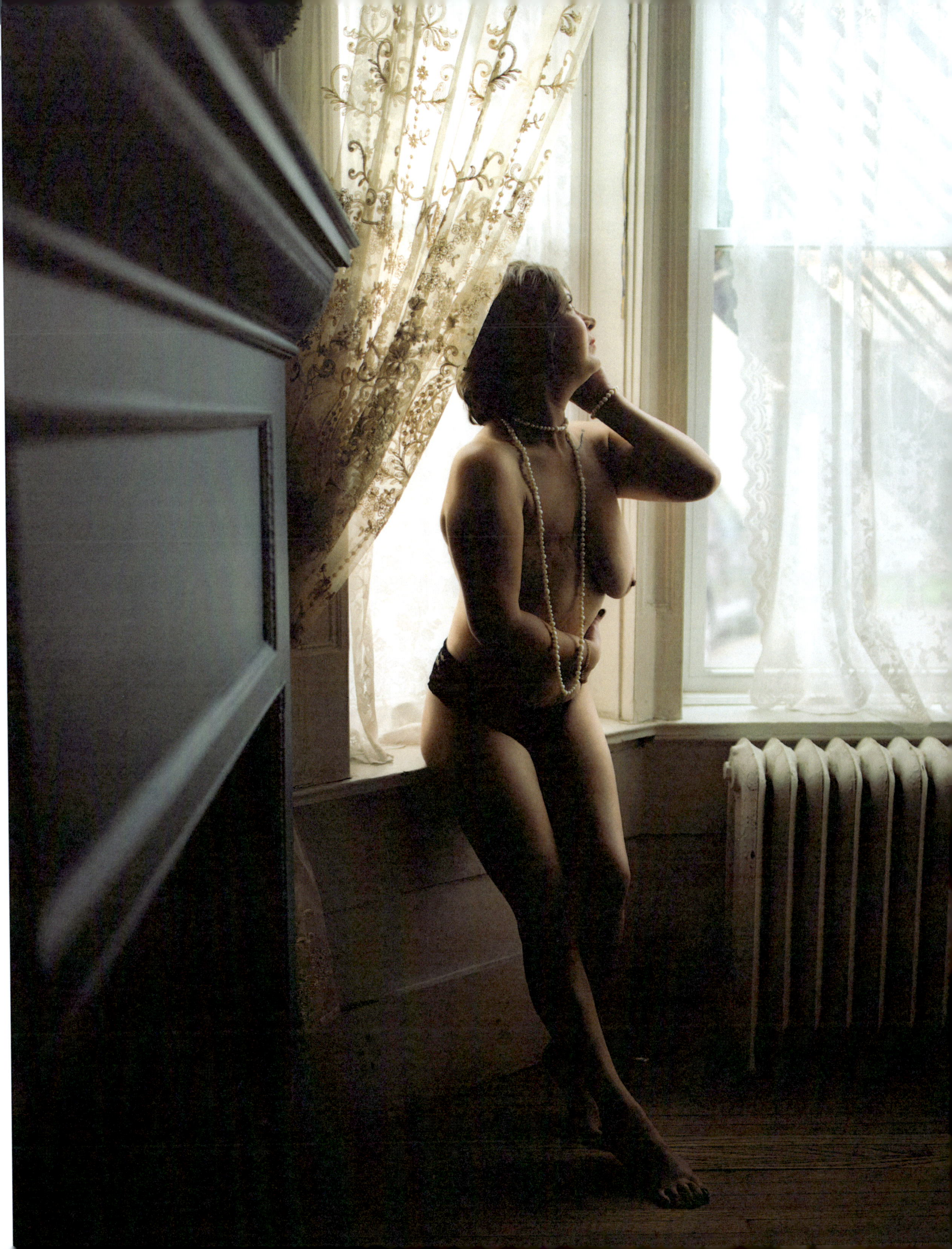

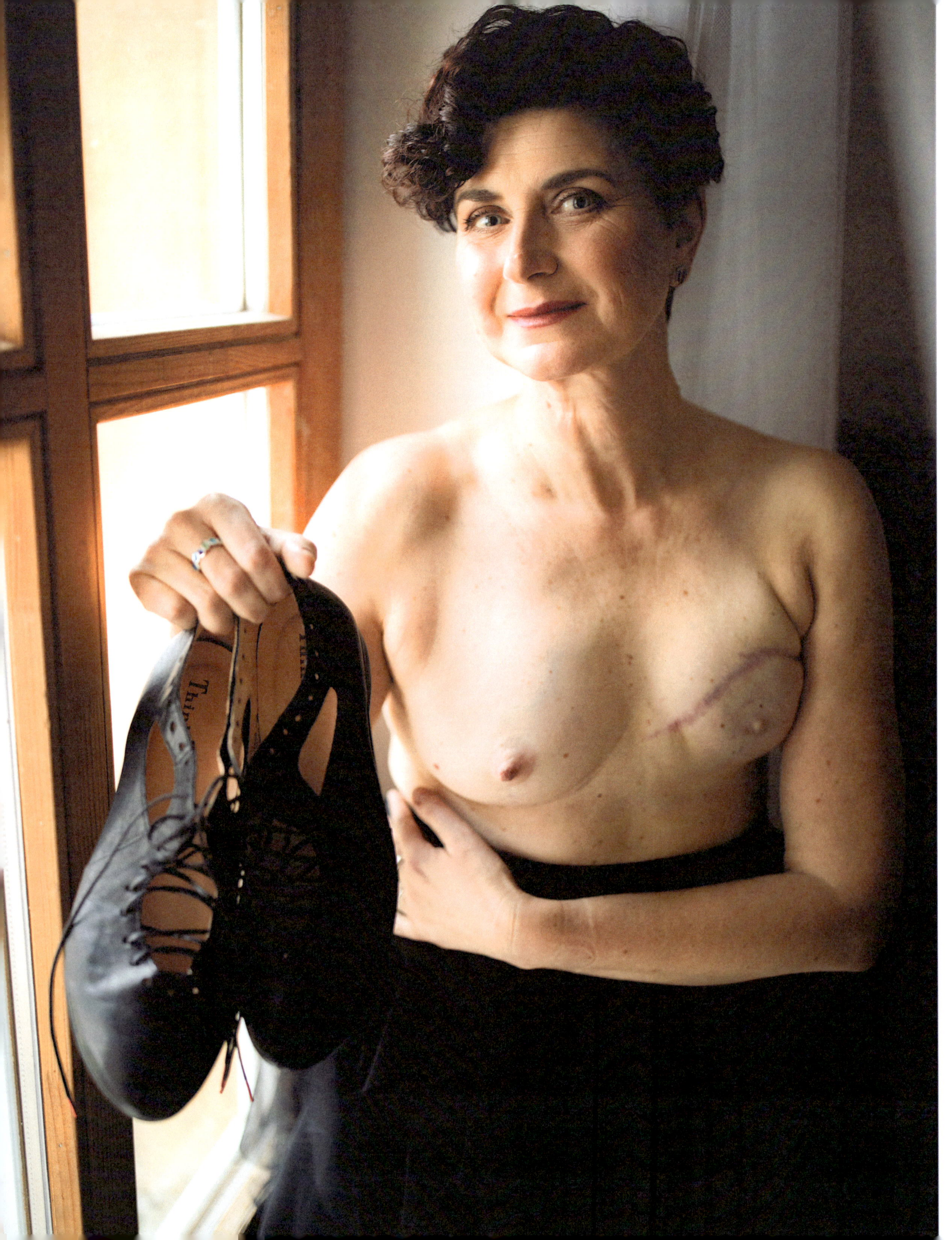

Diagnosis: *Breast Cancer, BRCA 1 gen.*
Age Diagnosed: *42*
Treatments Received: *Chemotherapy, mastectomy, breast implant.*
Age at time of photographs: *53*
Stage at time of photographs: *Remission*
Region: *Czech Republic*

I was 42 years old when I got cancer.

My daughter Vicky was 12 and my son Robin was 2.

The illness caught me off guard on the threshold of a new family life, after building a new home.

I didn't understand what was happening to me or why. But I bit my tongue and wanted to live. The idea of giving up never crossed my mind. Cancer was "just" an obstacle in the way. My doctor helped me by telling me the following "You are in for an unpleasant and difficult year. But there is a good chance of winning. I went through this myself with young children three years ago and fought through it. You can do it, you have the strength. You'll heal and you'll go on living. Some things are going to change, but you're just going to make it." It was very important for me to see and hear from someone who had survived the same diagnosis and was normally living and working.

I was very afraid of the surgery. I couldn't imagine how I'd live with a piece missing. But surprisingly, after the mastectomy came a huge relief that the tumor was gone. It just wasn't there, and I knew from the radiology that the cancer cells hadn't spread further into the nodes.

I was "clear" and it was a great feeling that gave me a lot of strength for my recovery.

My recommendation for life during and after cancer treatment is: have compassion for yourself and be kind to yourself. As much as you can. Reduce stress and demands on

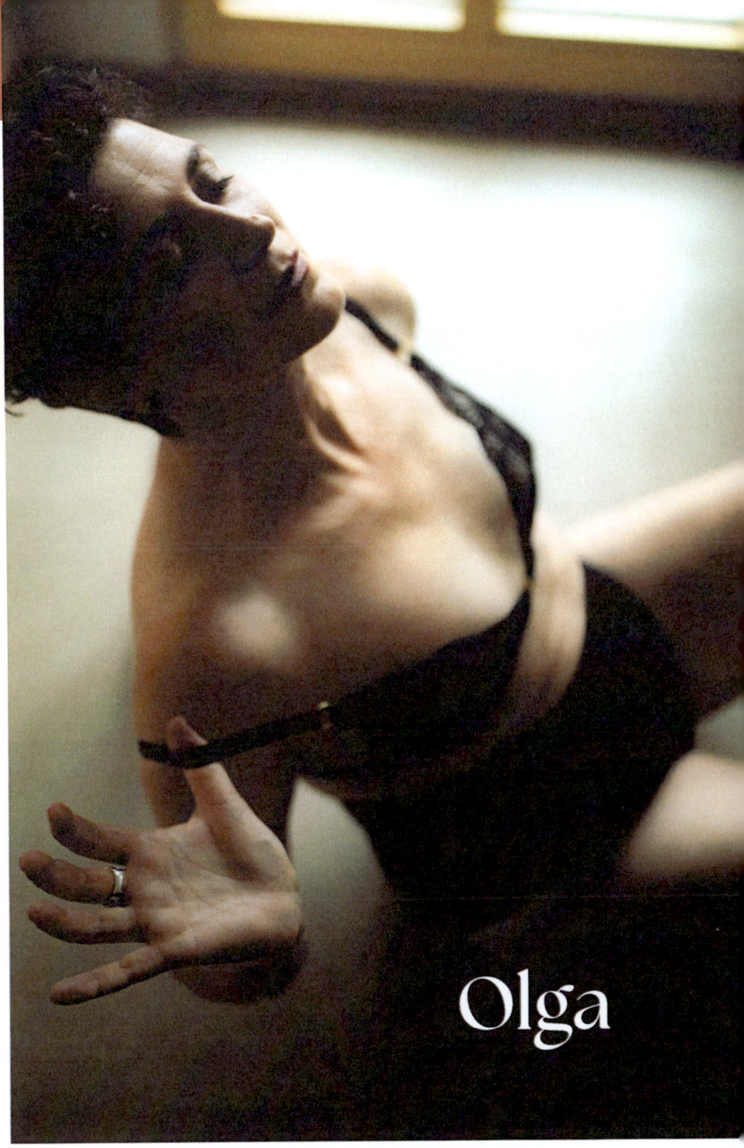

Olga

yourself. Don't be hard on yourself!

And if your treatment allows it then get outdoors, go to the mountains, ski, bike, work at least a little (if you enjoy work).

Rest, eat good food, enjoy every nice moment, and give up self-destructive habits.

From the perspective of my 55 year old self, I would add that a time of illness can be an amazing time of personal transformation. A time of redrawing your inner map.

And if you want to go down that road, I would seek out a therapist or a therapy group with whom you can share your deep fears and anxieties and then share with them also the progress on your journey.

Written, thought, and most importantly felt by Olga.🧡

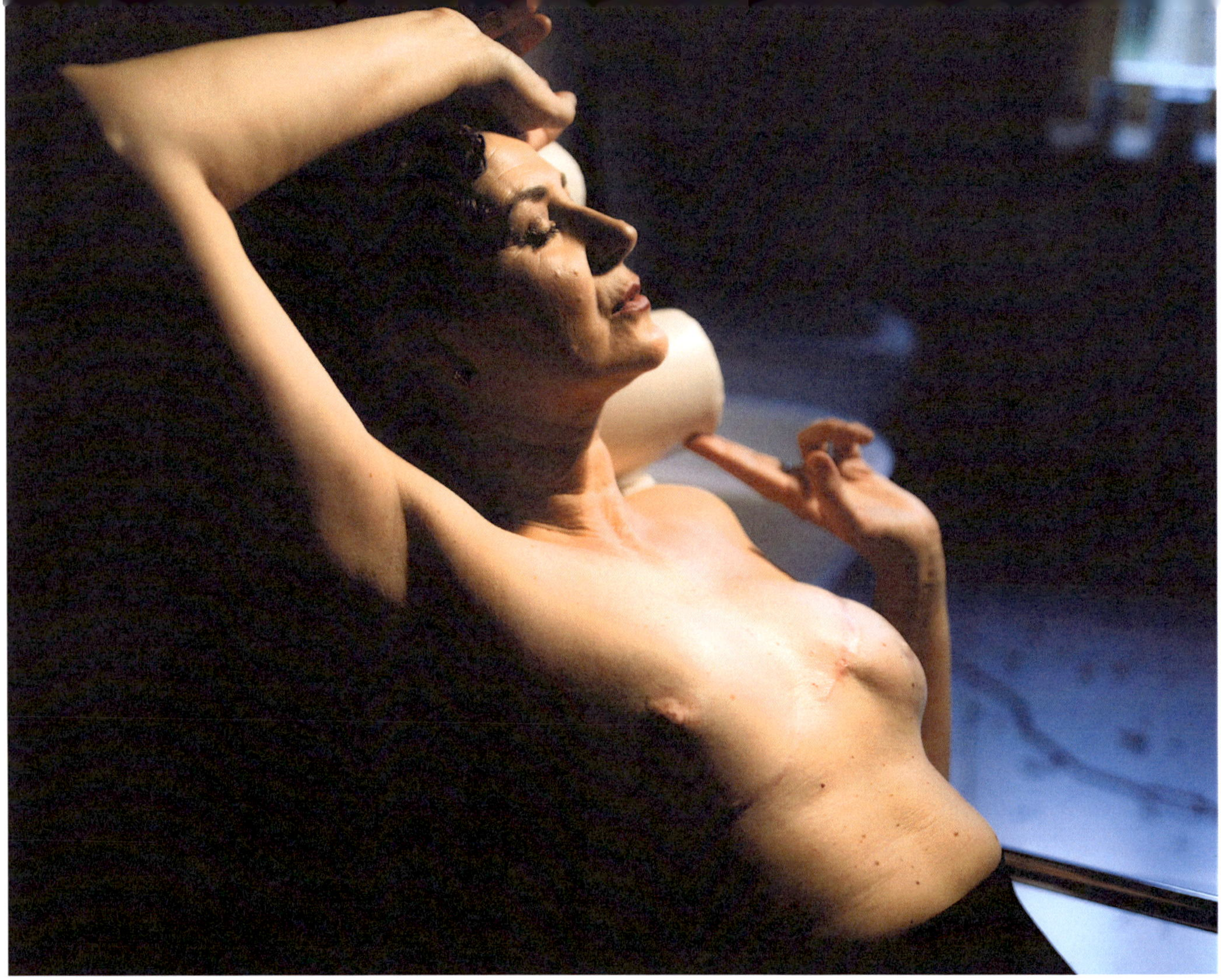

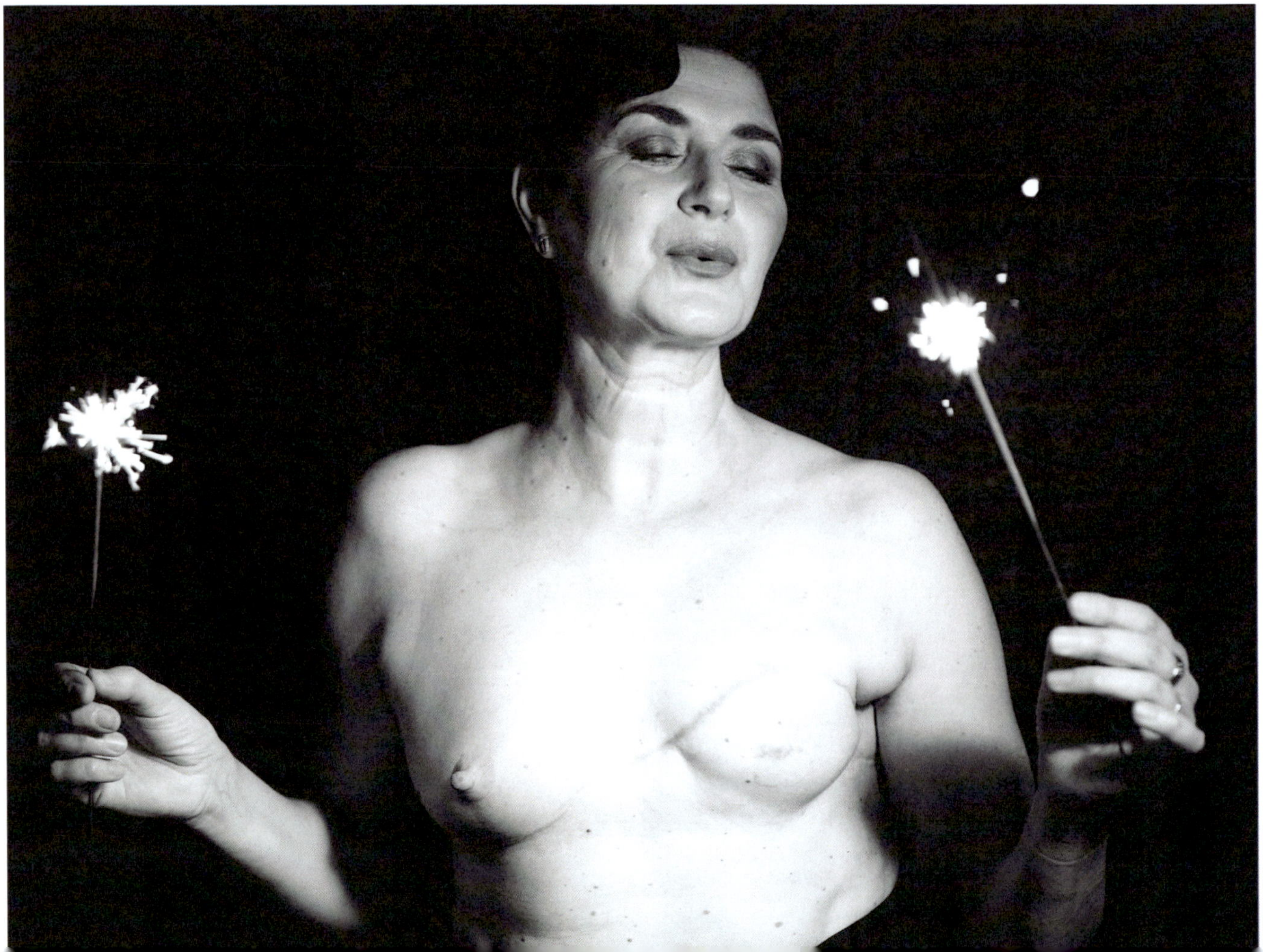

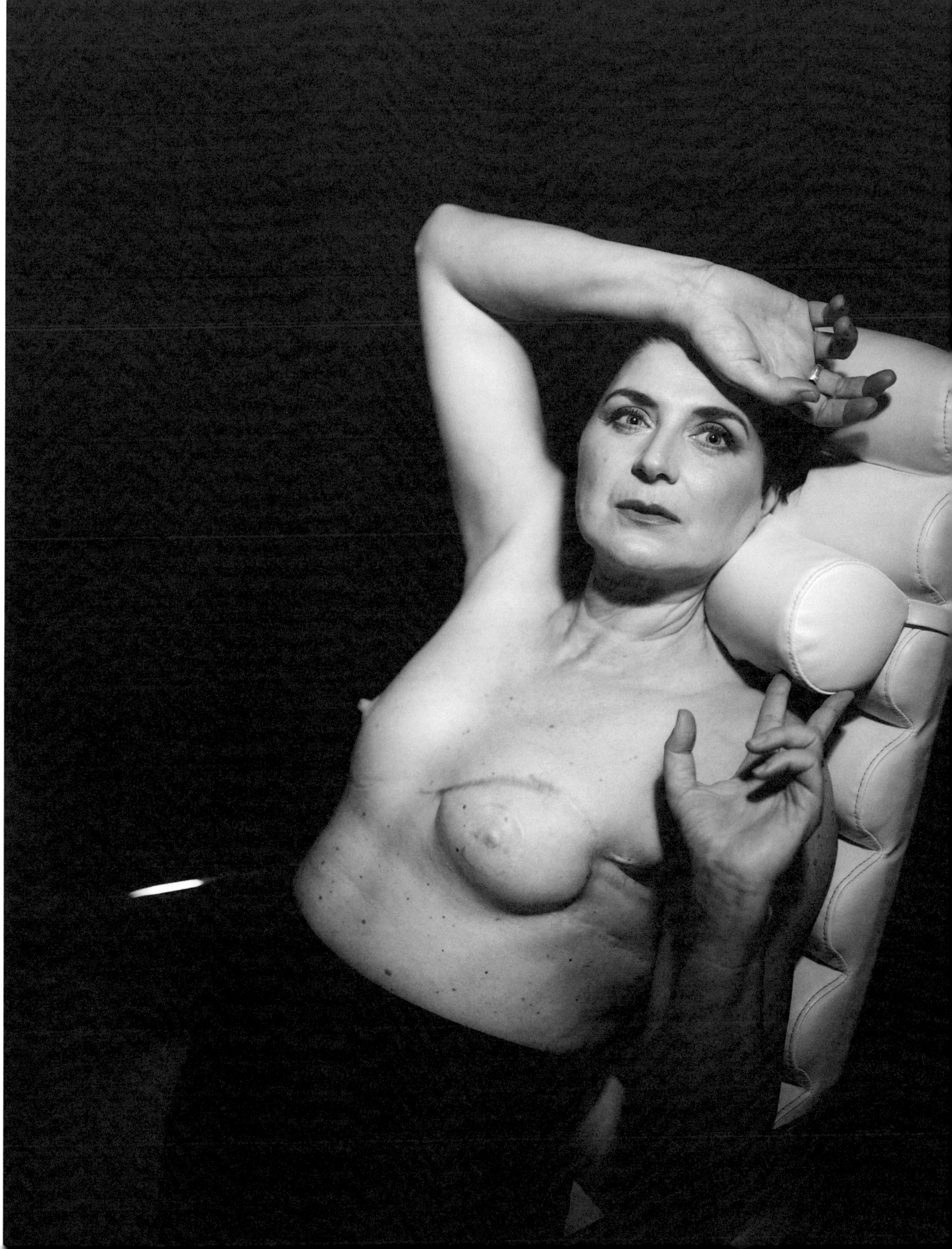

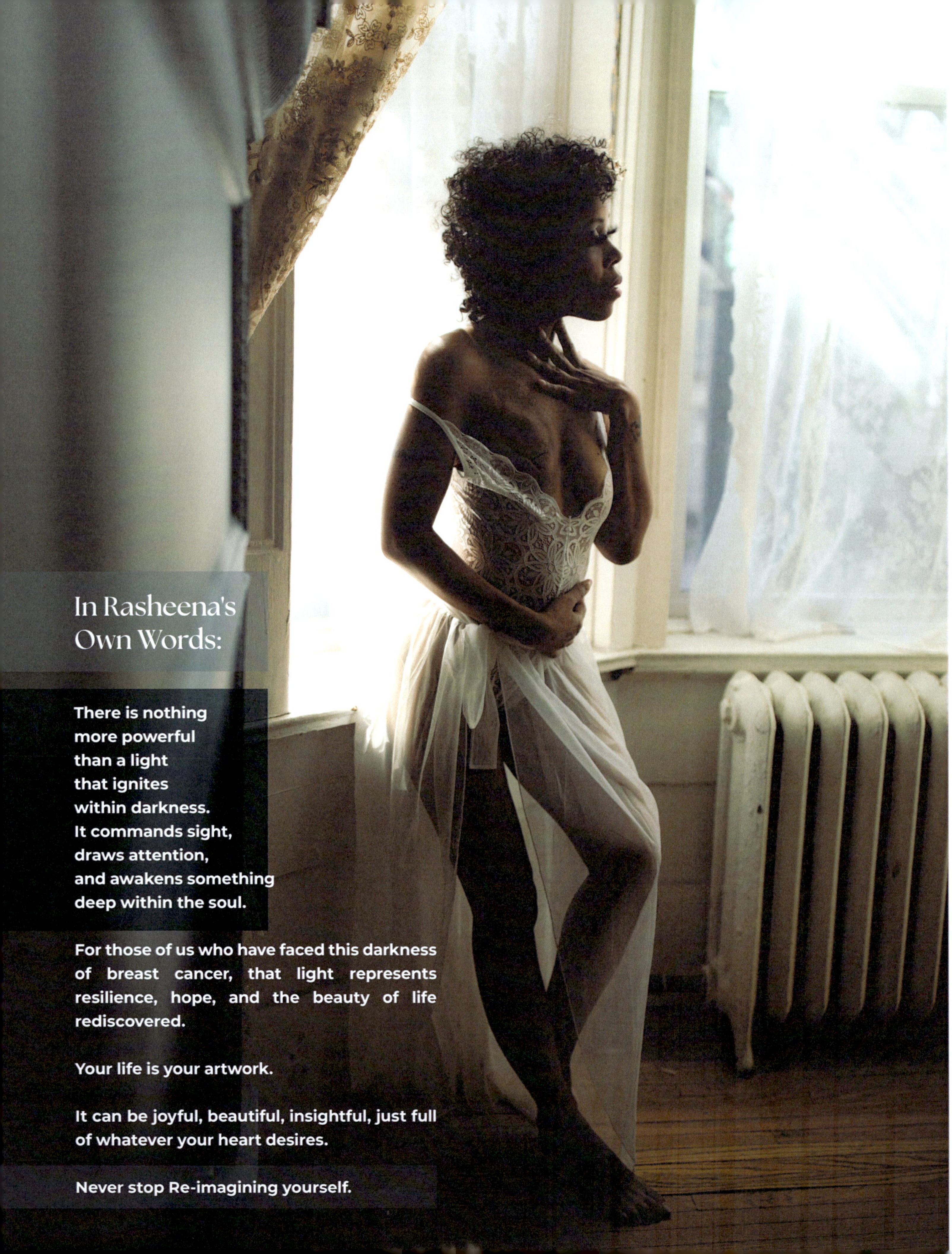

In Rasheena's Own Words:

There is nothing more powerful than a light that ignites within darkness. It commands sight, draws attention, and awakens something deep within the soul.

For those of us who have faced this darkness of breast cancer, that light represents resilience, hope, and the beauty of life rediscovered.

Your life is your artwork.

It can be joyful, beautiful, insightful, just full of whatever your heart desires.

Never stop Re-imagining yourself.

Diagnosis:	*Stage III Invasive Ductal Carcinoma*
Age Diagnosed:	*36 & recurrence at 38*
Treatments Received:	*Lumpectomy, Unilateral (single) Mastectomy, Chemotherapy, Immunotherapy*
Age at time of photographs:	*38*
Stage at time of photographs:	*Recently diagnosed with recurrence & metastatic disease*
Region:	*Philadelphia, PA*

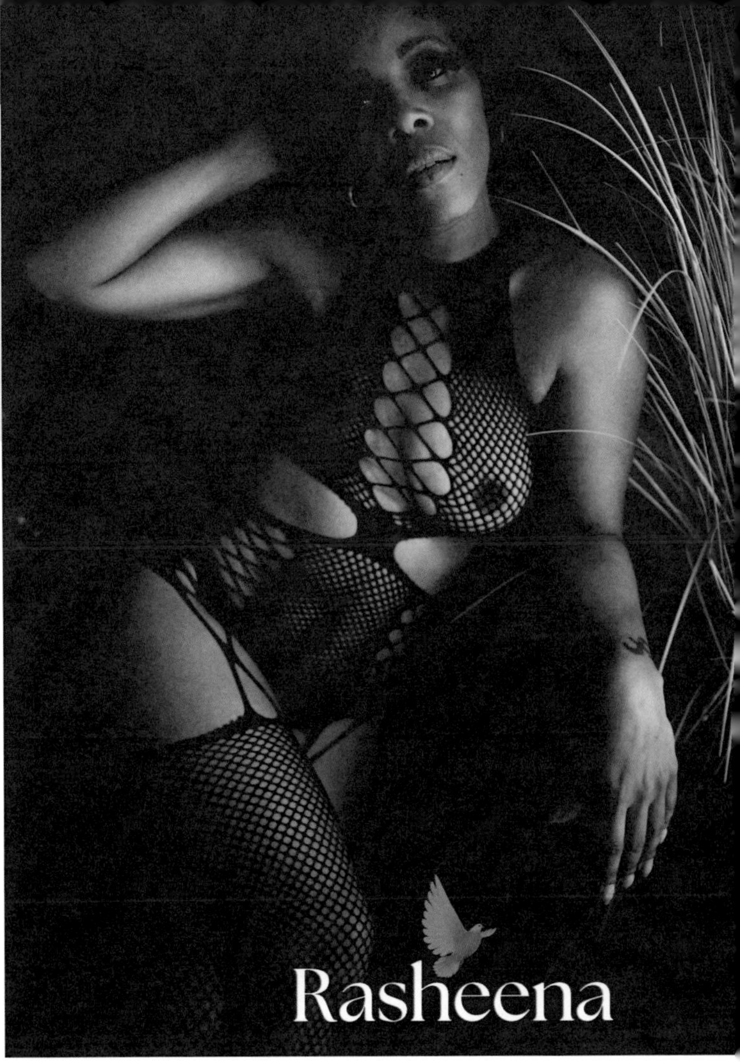

There was nothing quiet about the way that Rasheena Phinisee lived.

She was fierce. Intentional. Unafraid to speak hard truths, and unwilling to be overlooked. She was determined to be seen as a mother, an advocate, and someone who believed in joy even when things felt heavy. Her presence didn't just fill the room; it changed it.

She never planned to be silent about her diagnosis. In fact, she believed it was her responsibility to speak: to represent the lived experience of a Black woman navigating breast cancer, and to call attention to the disparities so many women of color face in the American healthcare system. She once told us "I feel it's part of my responsibility to represent black women with breast cancer." And she lived that truth with conviction.

Rasheena shared her story publicly and unapologetically. From the moment she felt a lump while breastfeeding her youngest daughter, which brought her to a crowded emergency room in the midst of a pandemic. That emergency room is where she met a concerned nurse who shifted her from dismissal to action. By the time she was diagnosed, the cancer had spread regionally.

Although treatment was difficult - after chemo, radiation, and a mastectomy, she experienced lasting damage to her lungs and bones - Rasheena never stopped giving. She kept thinking about others fighting similar battles while fighting her own. She created comfort kits for other women in treatment, packing them with things that could offer a moment of peace when everything felt overwhelming. She poured her heart into her charity Assiah's Liver Fund, and expanded it beyond her daughter's story to include breast health and support for women walking the same path. And through her podcast, Our Black Bodies, she opened space for raw, necessary conversations about race, illness, and what it means to reclaim your body when the world and the system have tried to take it from you.

Rasheena's story is not defined by her death in August 2024, but by her fierce presence while she lived. She was a mother of three, including a teen daughter who had received two liver transplants, and a toddler on the autism spectrum. She was a fierce advocate, a builder of community, and a woman who demanded better from the system - not just for herself, but for everyone else it too often fails.

Though she passed before she could submit her piece for this book, her voice remains powerful and clear. It's in the words she spoke, the lives she touched, the systems she challenged, and the stories she made room for. Rasheena believed deeply in the importance of visibility and representation, and she embodied that belief with grace and grit.

This space in You Are Whole is for her. For her power. Her legacy. And her insistence that every story, especially those too often overlooked, deserves to be told.

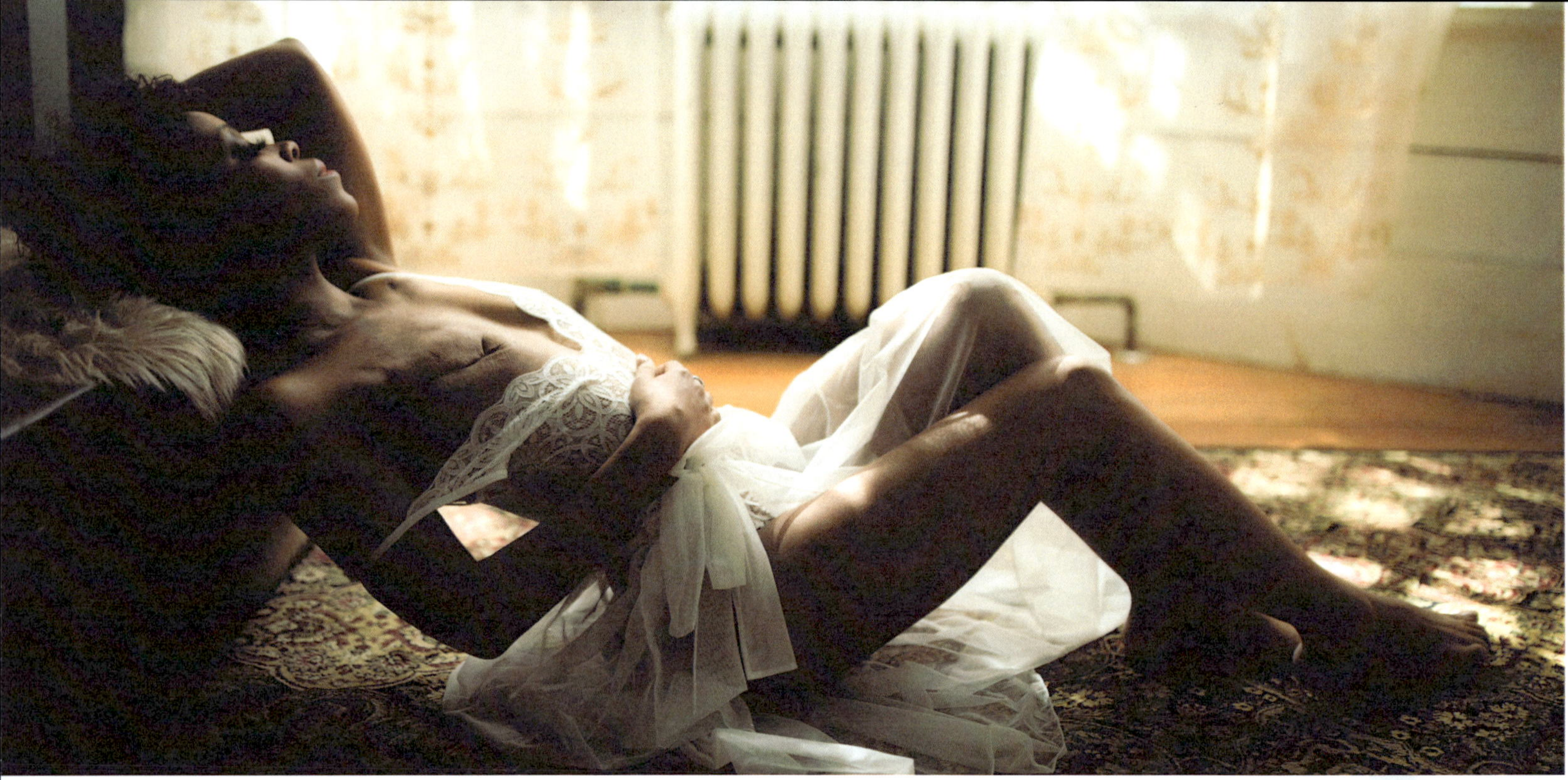

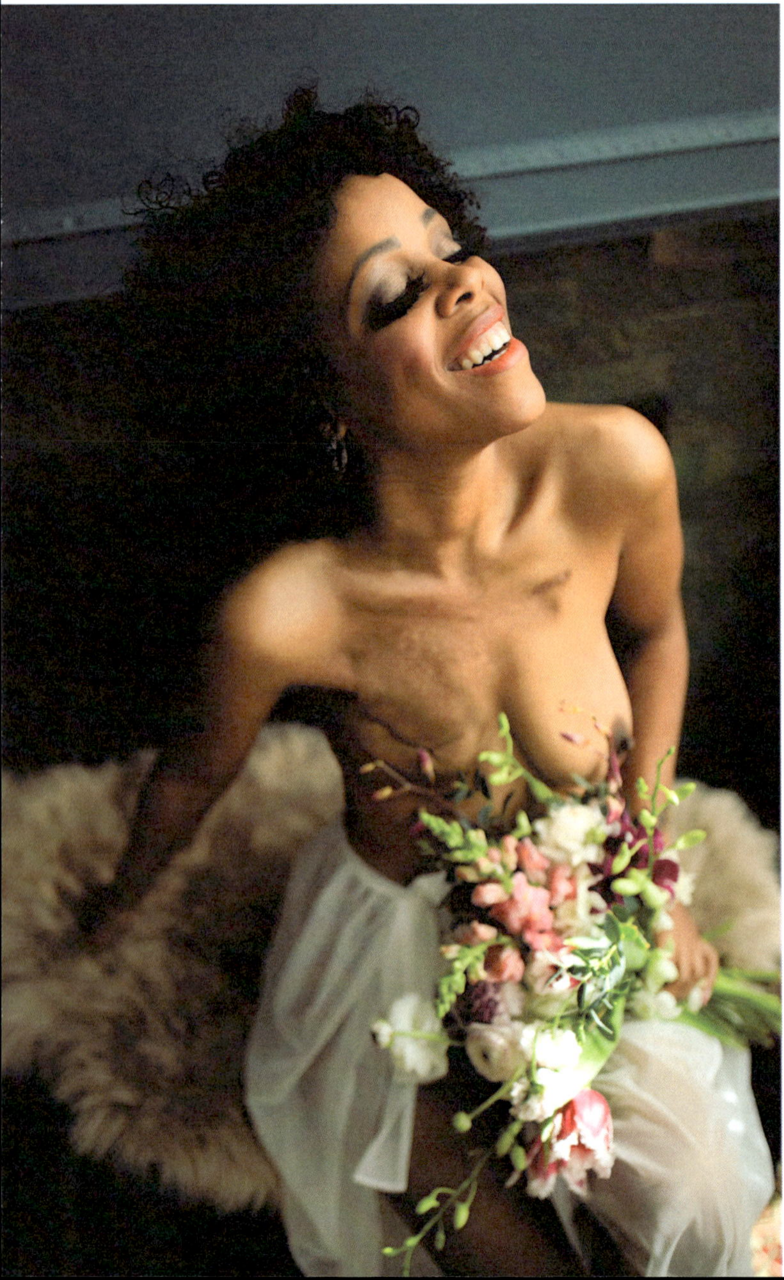

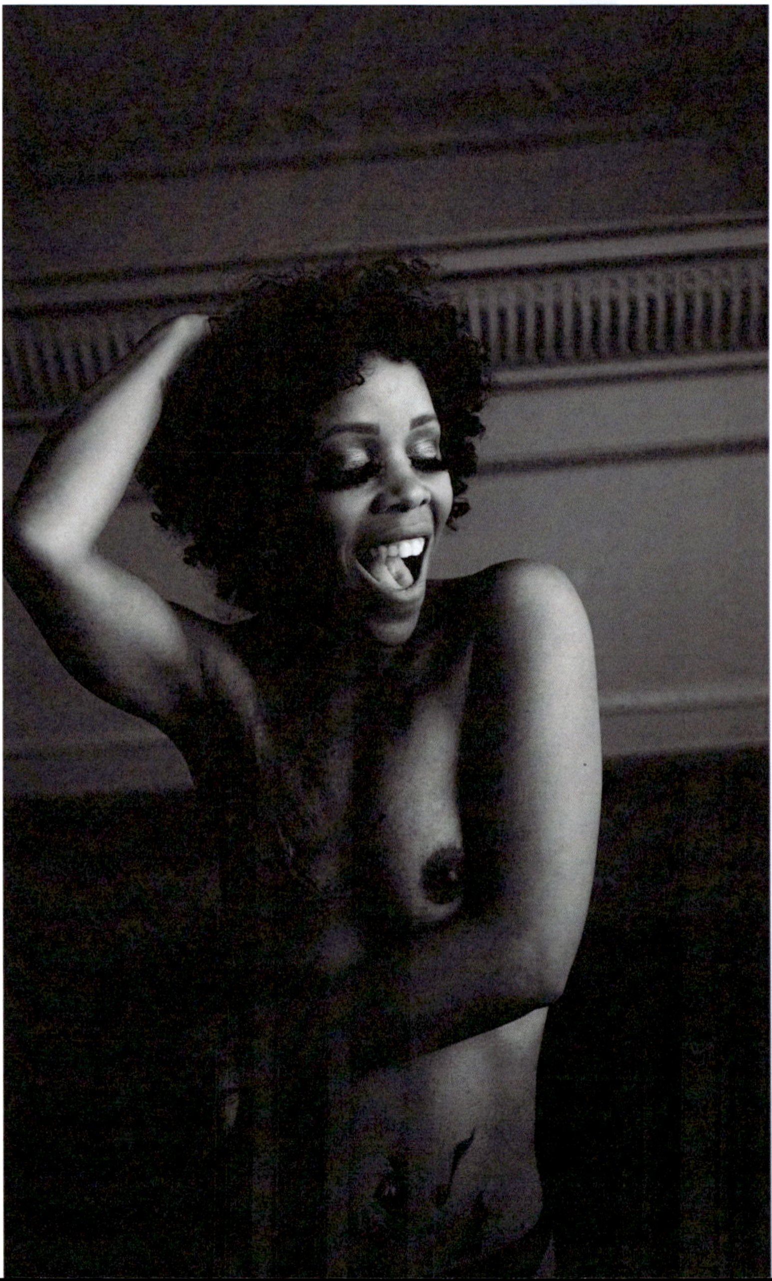

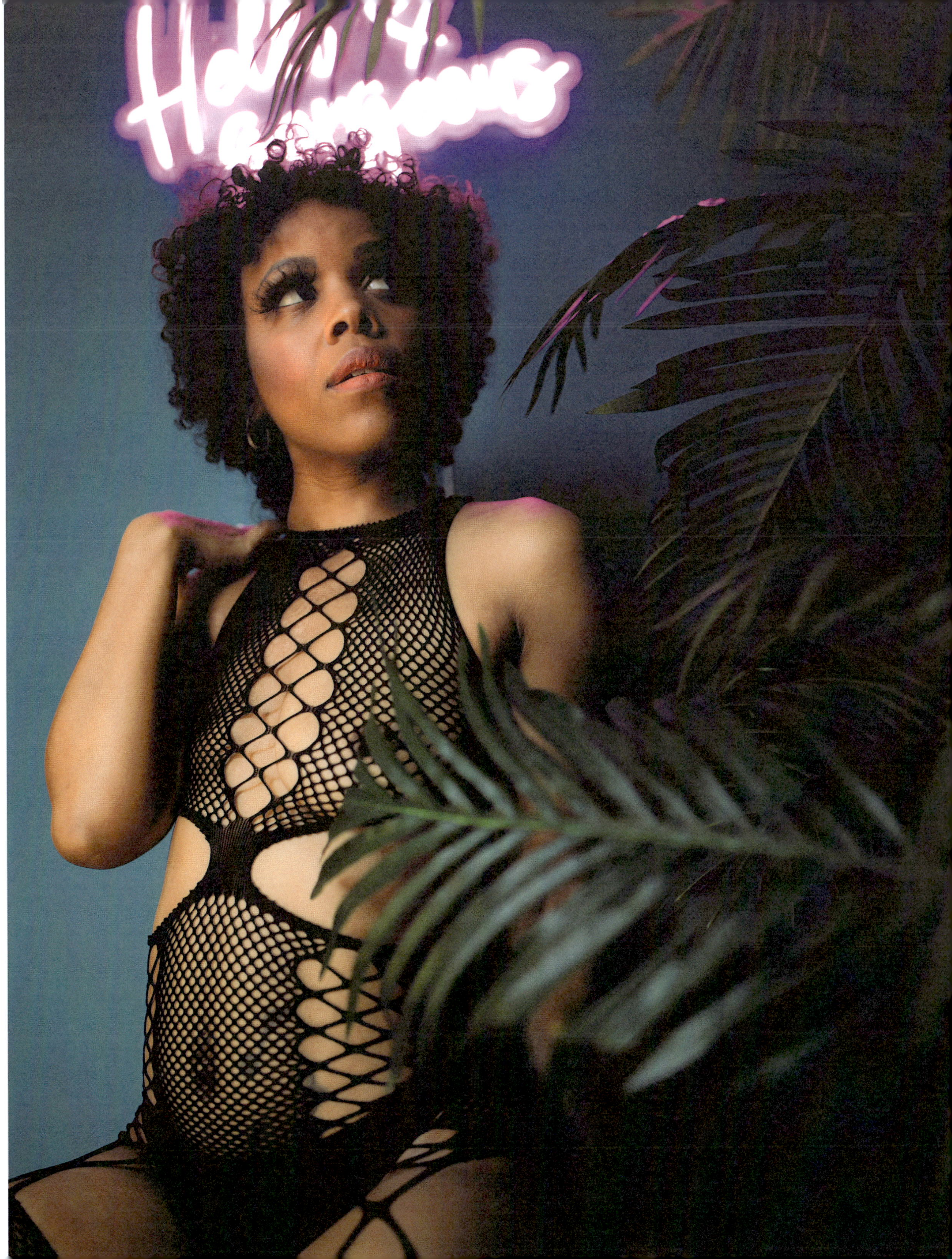

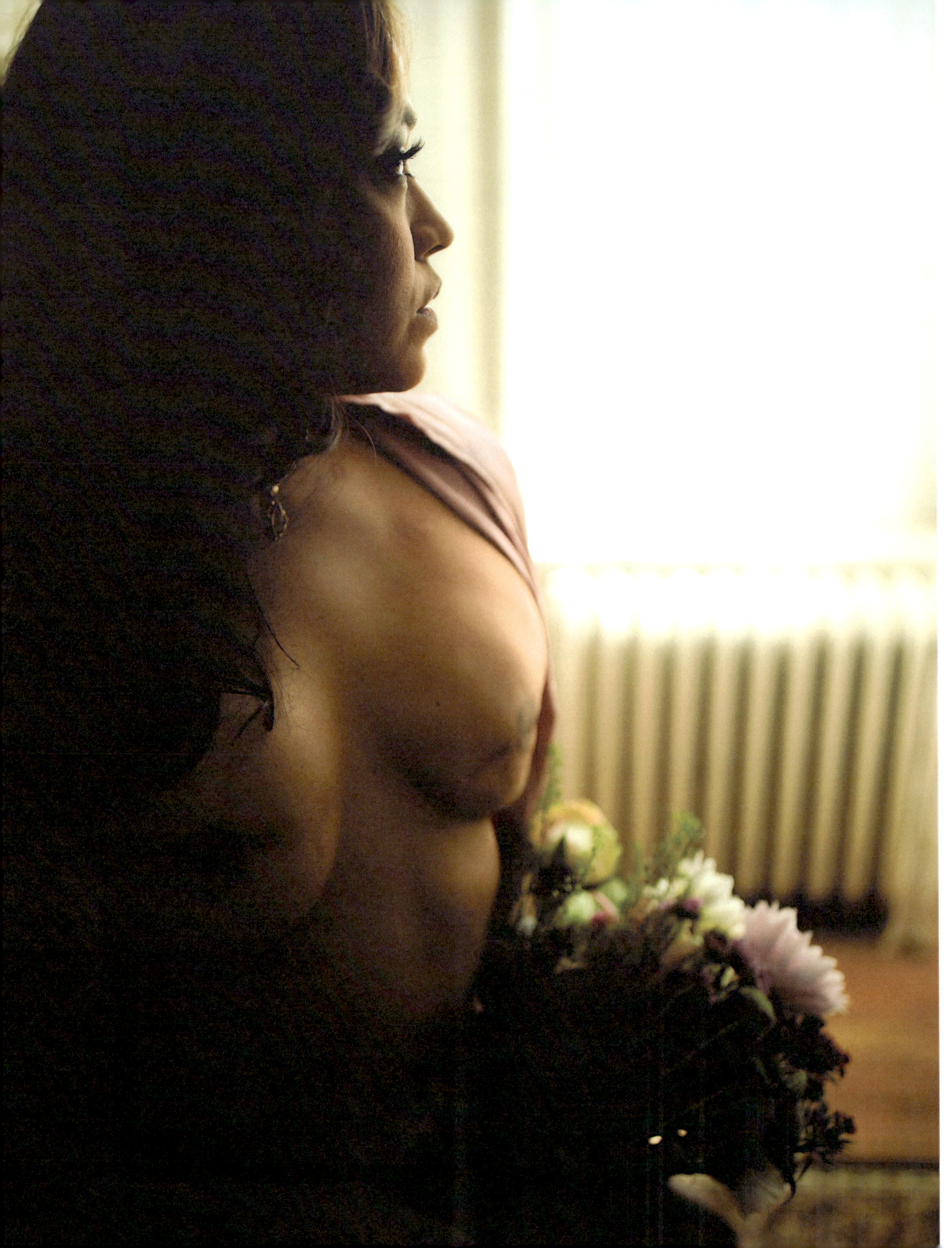

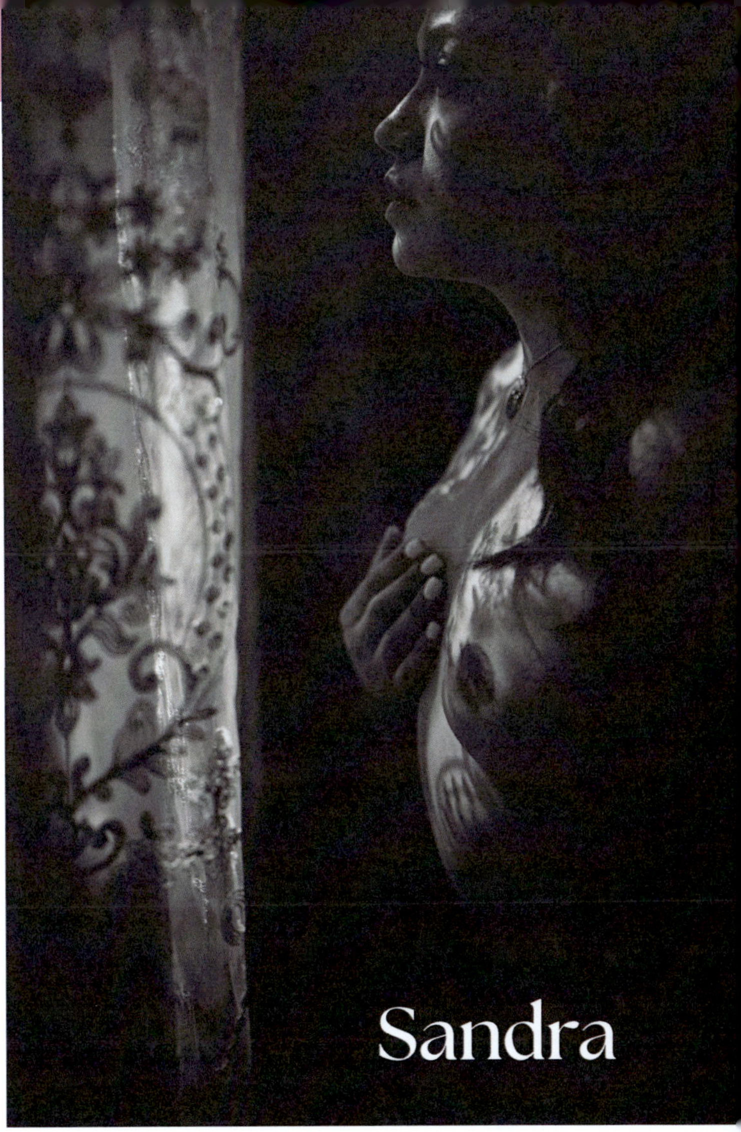

Sandra

Diagnosis:	Invasive Ductal Carcinoma Stage 3b estrogen&proges+ her2-
Age Diagnosed:	34
Treatments Received:	Bilateral mastectomy with 2 reconstruction surgeries (one corrective), 16 weeks of chemotherapy (A,C,T drugs), 5 and 1/2 weeks of radiation, IVF treatment, chest port placement twice, Bone infusions for 5 years, lupron shots every 3 months for a total of 10 years, daily oral medication for 10 years.
Age at time of photographs:	38
Stage at time of photographs:	4 years in remission
Region:	Massachusetts

I have been self-conscious of my body since I was a young girl.

The relationship between my body and weight was even more negatively impacted after moving to the USA.

Once diagnosed, the reality of accepting that you have no control of what your body is doing during treatment while being ok and wanting to stay alive was a lot to manage. The struggle of barely recognizing yourself and not being able to stare in the mirror. I spent many days hating my body for what it was doing but at the same time grateful that I was alive. All the self-confidence I had was out of the window and I felt lost most of the time. I did not think I could overcome it.

The one thing that kept me going was my body and the fact that it did not want to give up. Closer to the end of my treatments and corrective surgeries, I felt a strong disassociation with my body.

The daily struggle of appreciating being alive and staring at your scars while feeling lost inside your own body became a battle for years to come. I started walking outdoors and doing small hikes which brought me some happiness I was searching for. I felt more "normal" for a lack of a better word and my self-love and self-care was growing in me. I gained a little fire inside of me that told me I was doing things right, to keep going.
The day came of the photoshoot and all the doubts flooded my body and mind. I felt like I was going to bomb and that I just would not be able to deliver because of the body dysmorphia that I felt at that very moment.

Seeing my photos, I did not recognize the girl in the camera. I felt this immense sense of power and strength building inside of me. I felt warm, confident, sexy, and powerful all at the same time. For this moment I realized there is nothing wrong with me and with my body. I am beautiful and whole just as I am here, the survivor who fought breast cancer and won.

I gained my confidence and felt a deep sense of love and self-compassion. I know that not every day is great, but I always remind myself how much of a badass you must be, to beat this and still thrive.

My takeaway from my own experience has been to be kind to myself and my body and to always acknowledge that each day is a new day to love yourself more all over again because you deserve it.

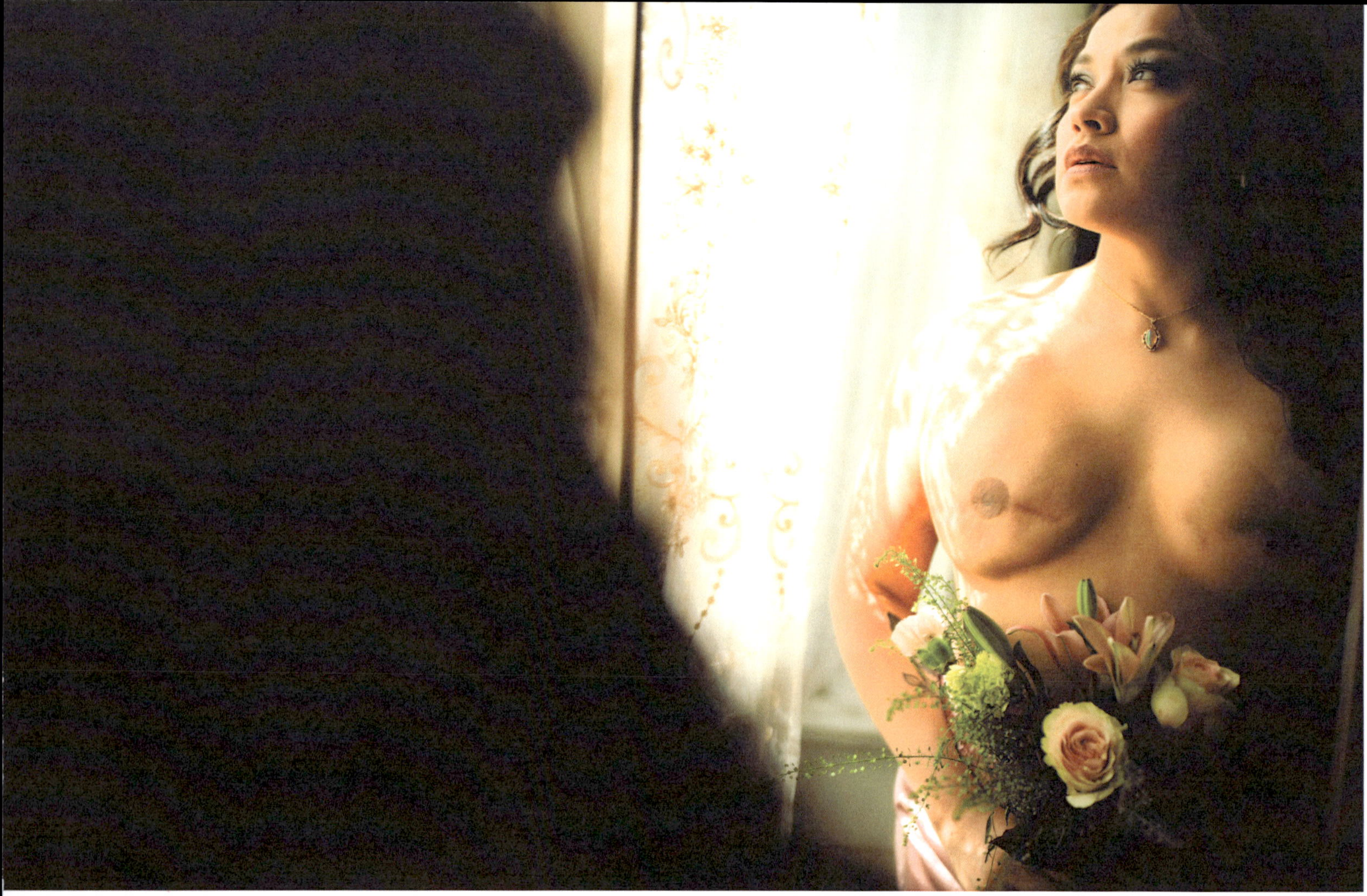

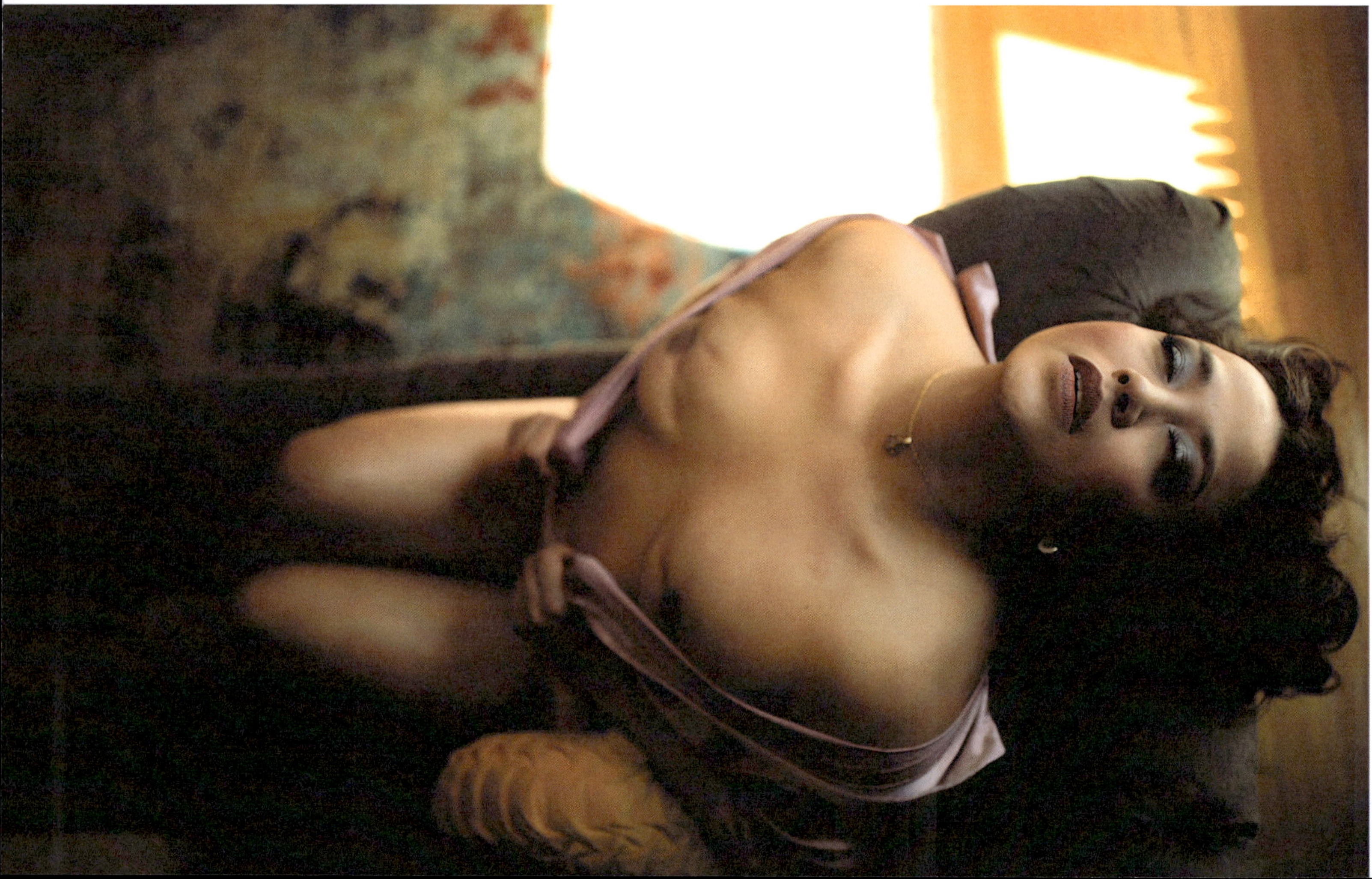

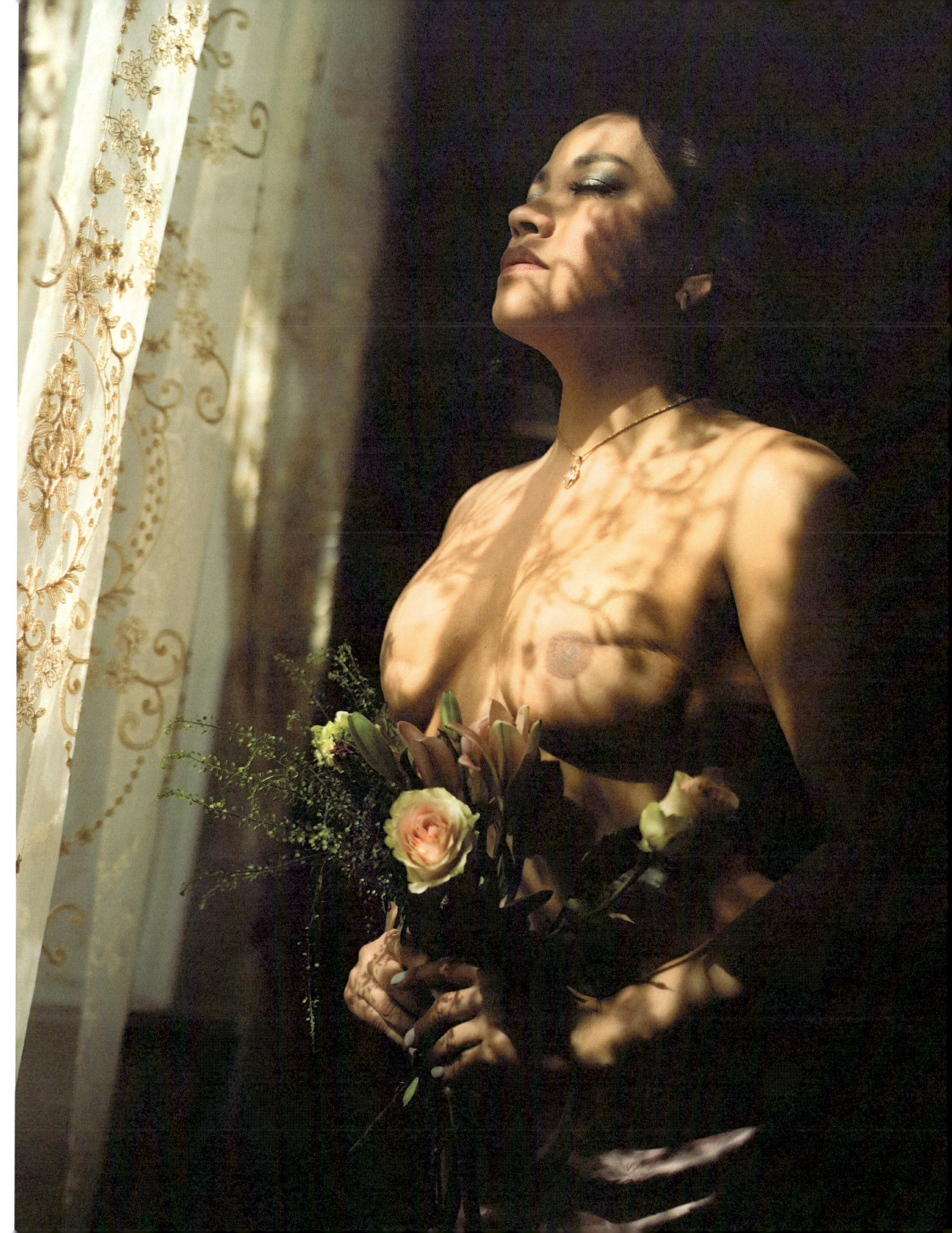

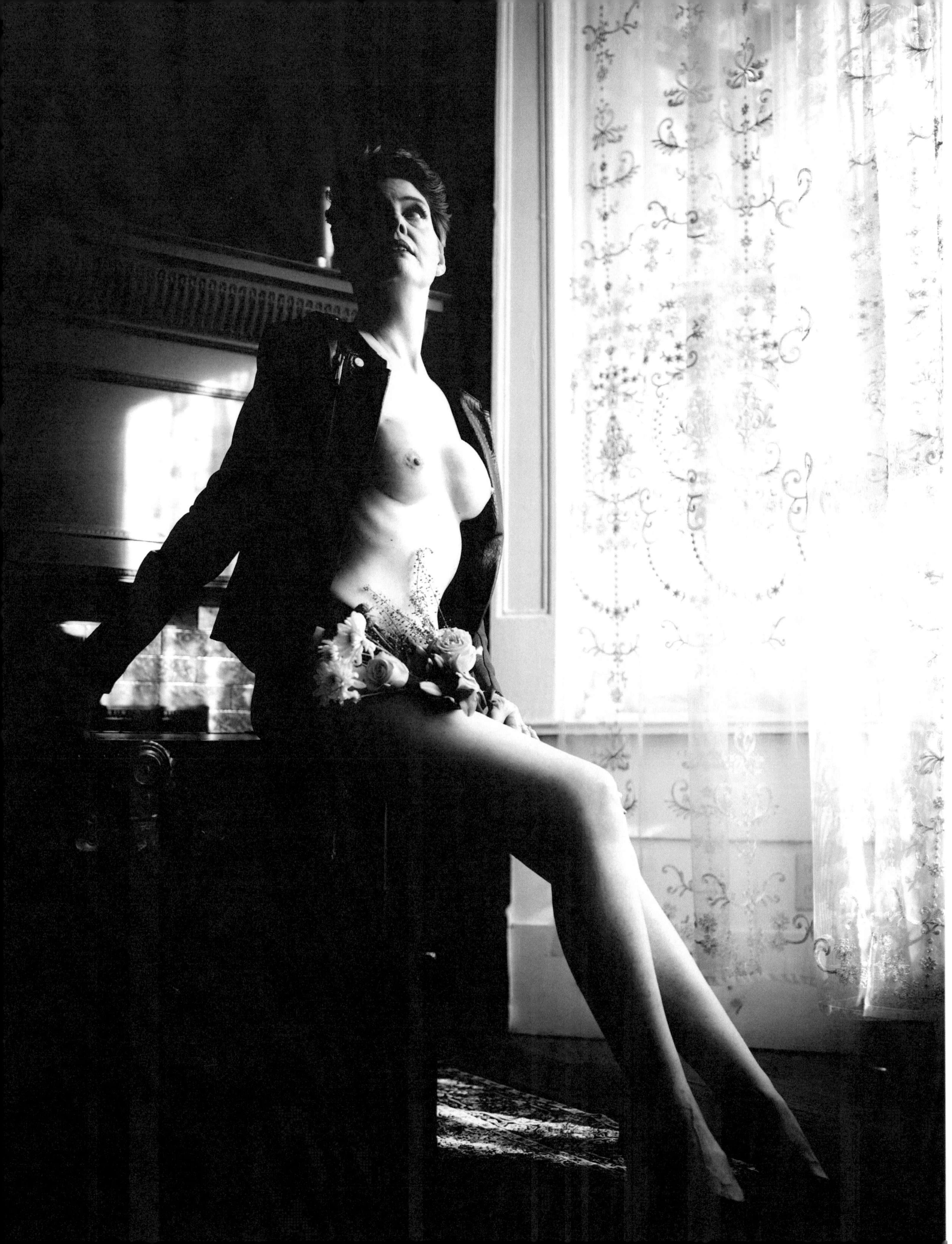

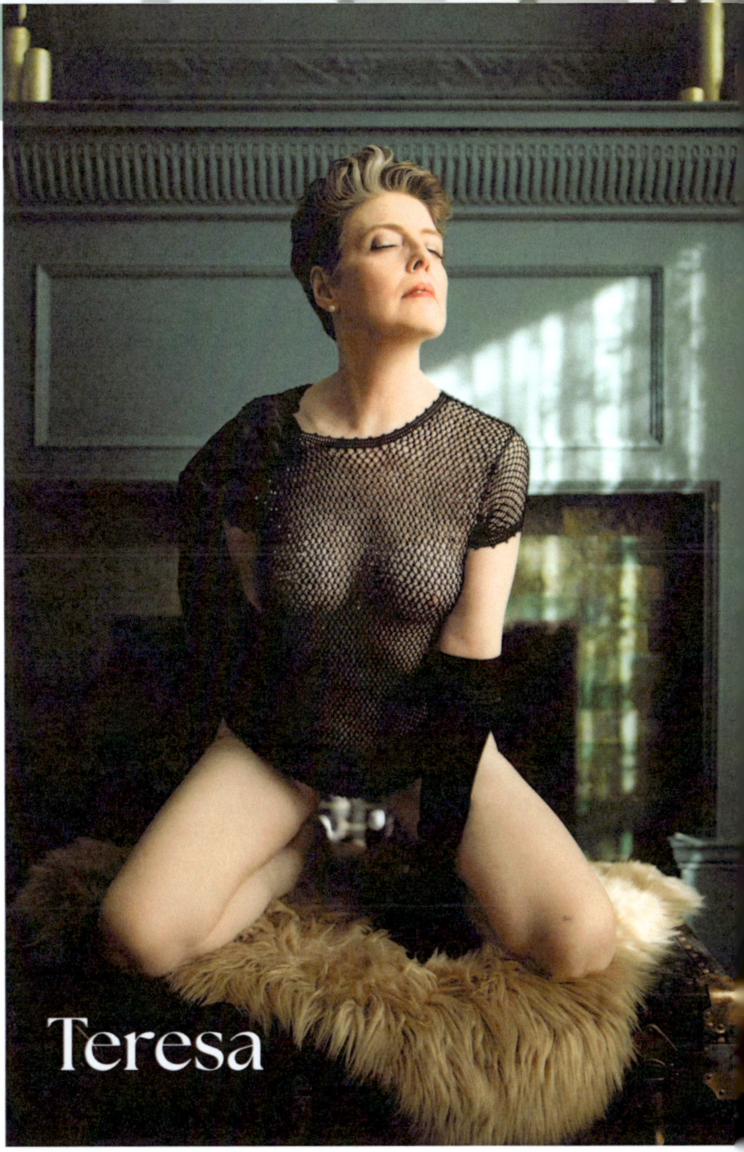

Diagnosis: *Invasive Ductal Carcinoma HR+ HER2-, PALB2 mutation.*
Age Diagnosed: *53*
Treatments Received: *Double Mastectomy, Chemotherapy, Radiation, Hormone Therapy.*
Age at time of photographs: *55*
Stage at time of photographs: *Stage III*
Region: *Northeast*
Social Media: *@newyorknolan*

Cancer is a strange and unpleasant experience.

I do not recommend it.

But if you must go through it, here is what I think you should know:

Cancer changes you. Initially, and maybe for some time, you will want to go back to your old life, the old you, but you can't, not really.

The disease forges you, like steel in the fire. It is difficult, sometimes exceedingly so.

It can be mentally taxing, physically challenging, emotionally devastating.

But you do it.

You take one step at a time.

You listen to your doctors, but most of all you listen to yourself, your body, your gut.

You breathe!

As you go through all of it, you may come to realize how lucky you are to be alive and that there is no time to waste on insecurity, on competition, on small stuff.

You appreciate the beauty of nature and the small, quiet moments much more than before. You allow yourself to feel everything you feel.

You cry.

You grieve.

You accept help.

You move your body.

You connect with others like yourself.

You accept your new body and all the changes with love.

You remind yourself that you are your own best friend.

You recognize that you have more confidence than before.

You realize how powerful and courageous you really are.

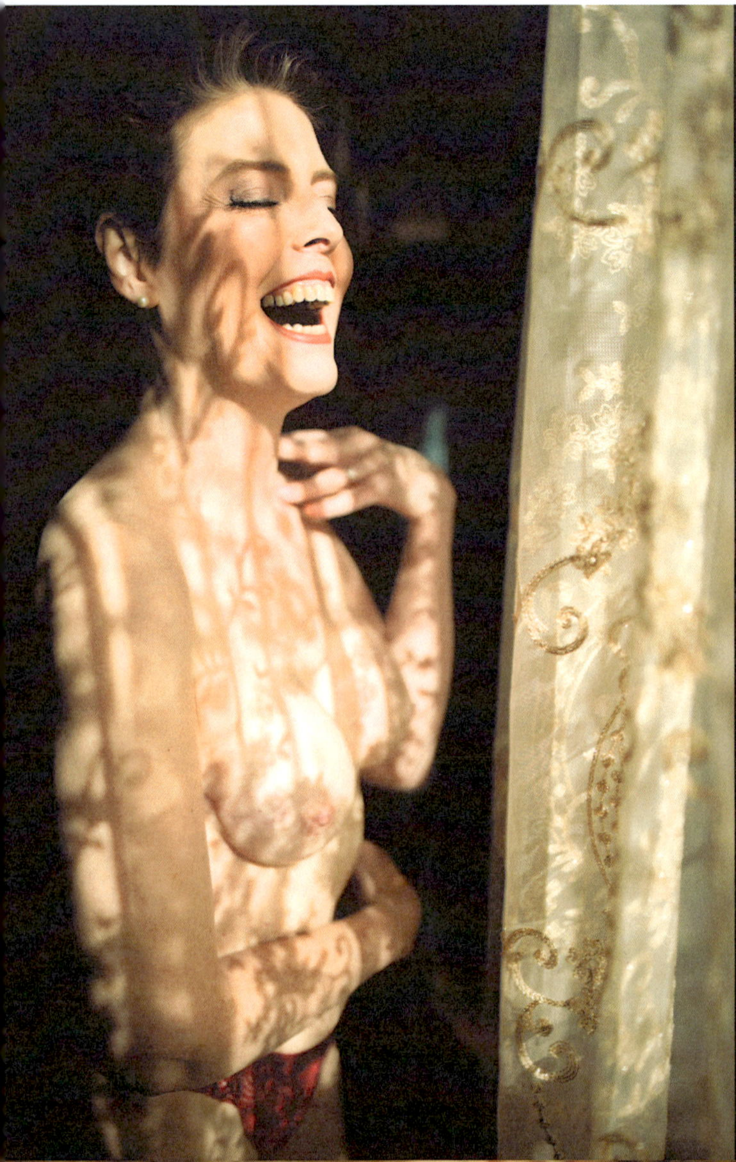
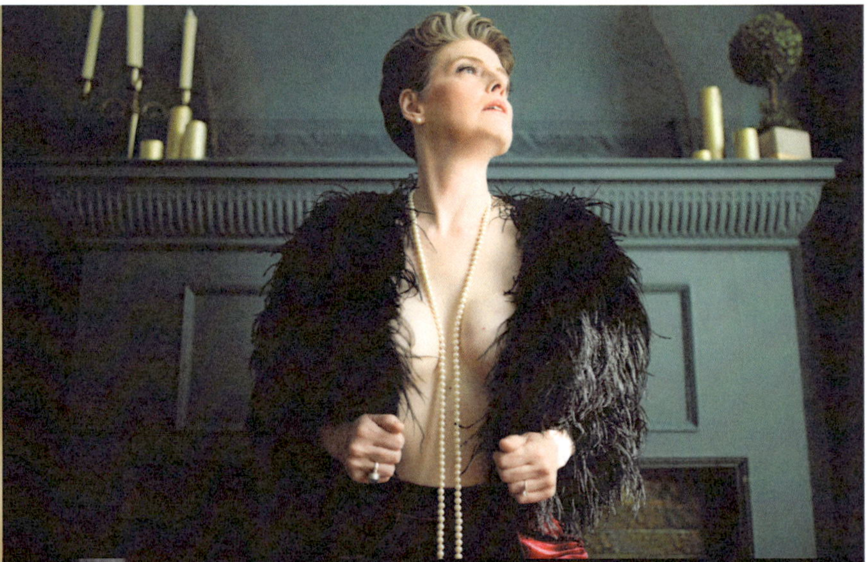
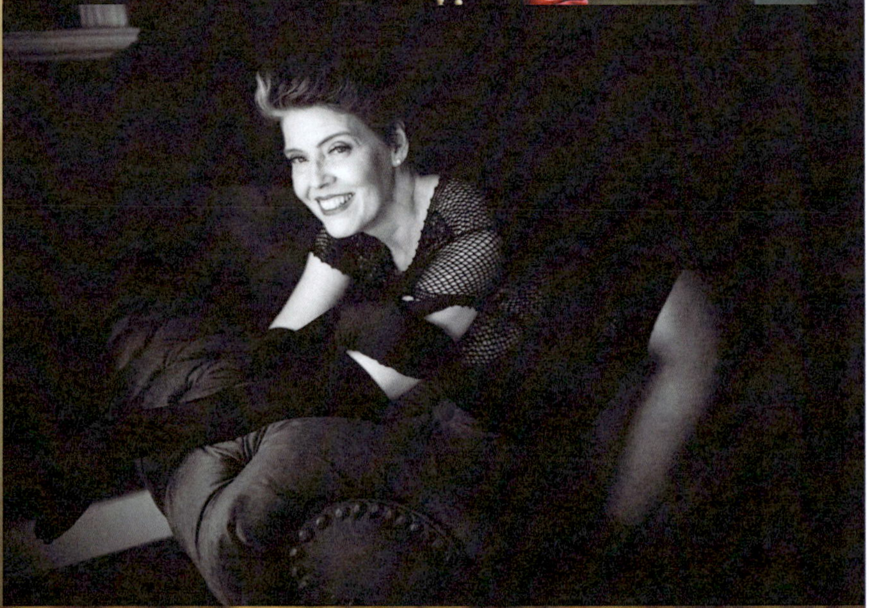
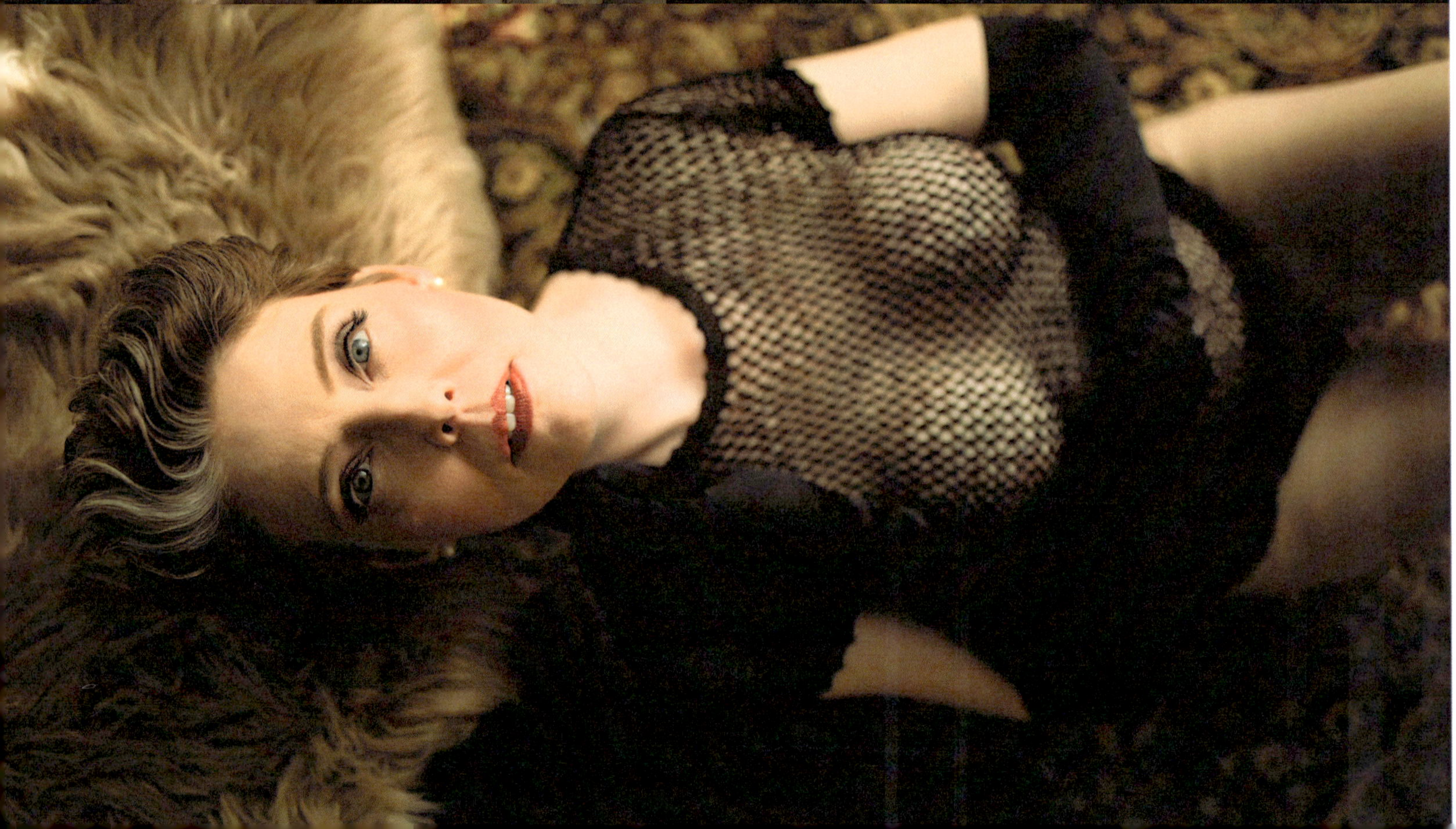

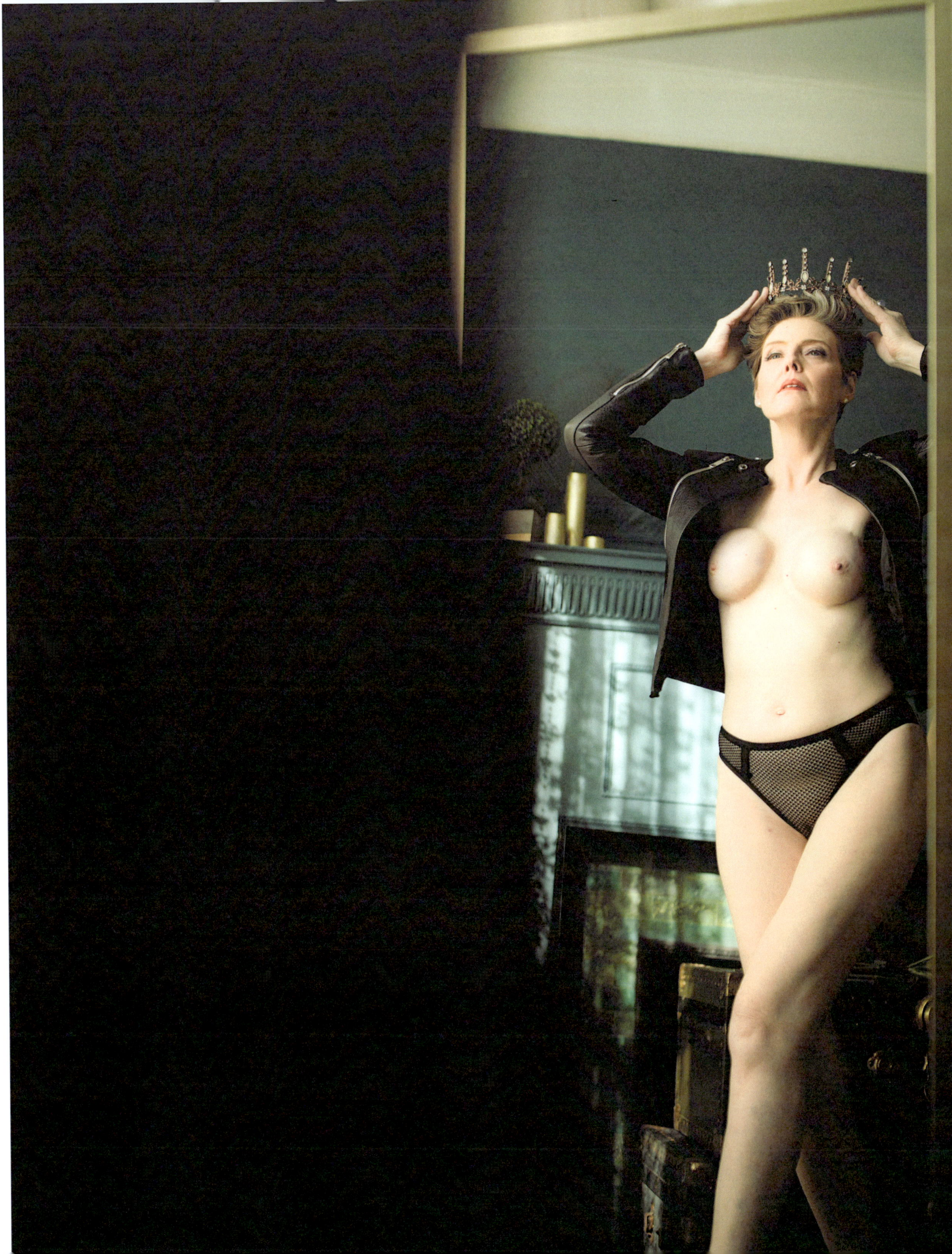

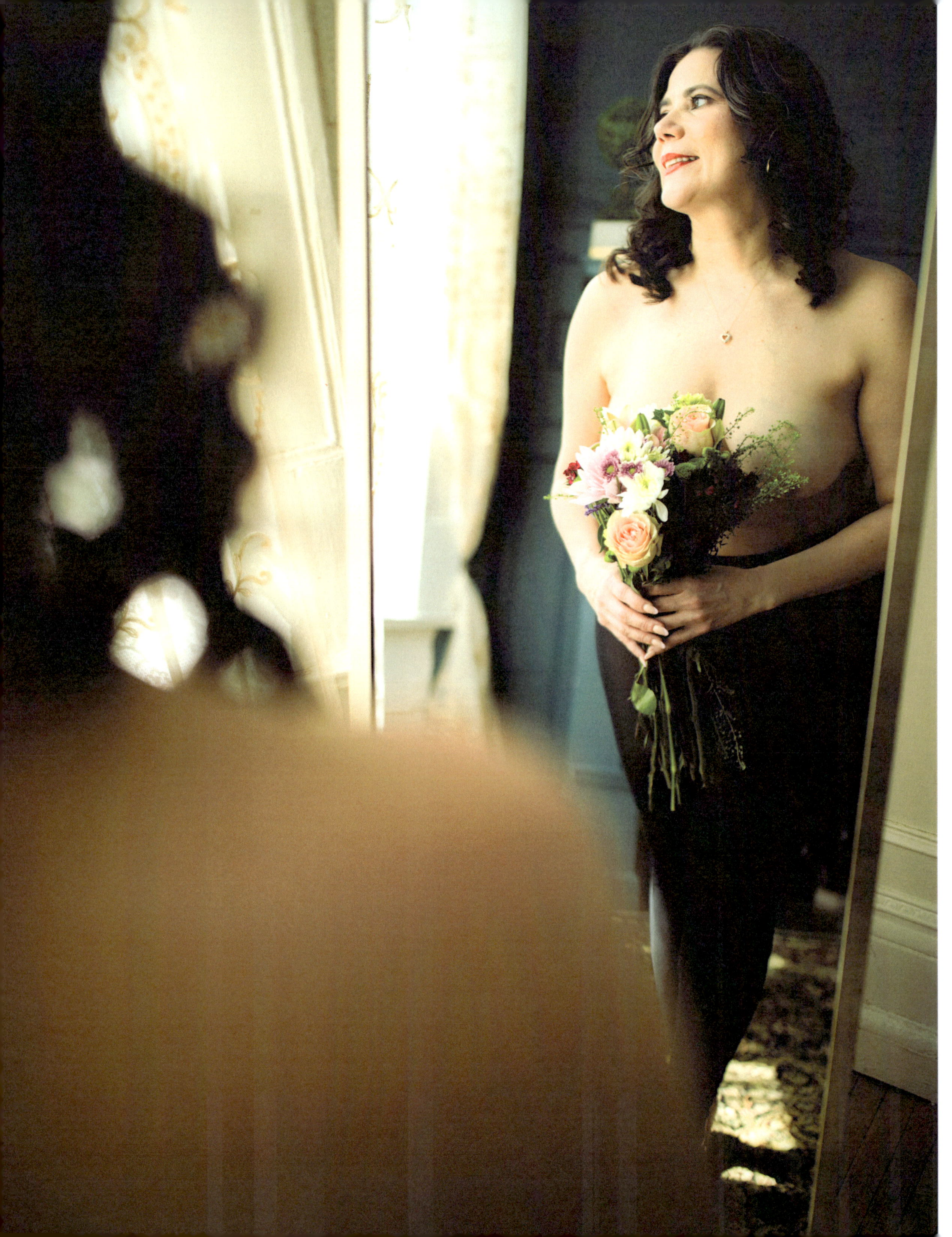

Diagnosis: *Invasive Ductal Carcinoma (IDC), estrogen Receptors positive (ER+), progesterone Receptors positive (PR+)*
Age Diagnosed: *43*
Treatments Received: *Lumpectomy, radiation therapy and Tamoxifen.*
Age at time of photographs: *48*
Stage at time of photographs: *4th year remission*
Region: *New York*

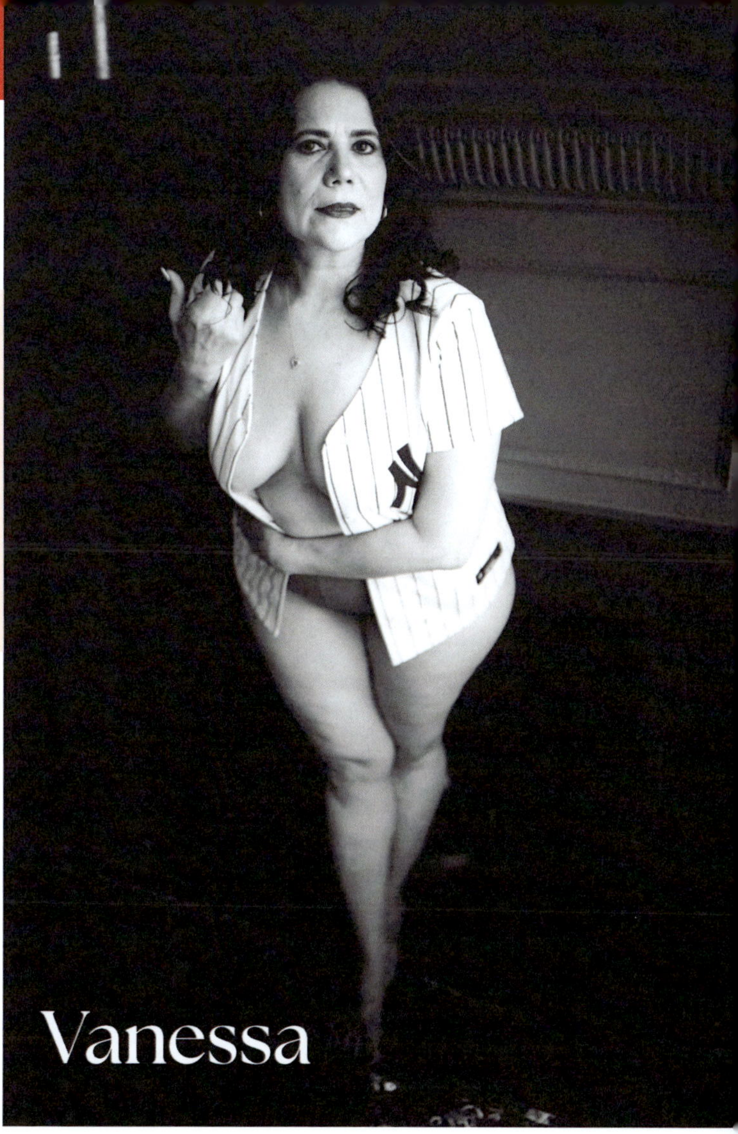

Vanessa

I was diagnosed during Breast Cancer Awareness month in 2019, how ironic, on a routine check.

I felt most vulnerable after my second biopsy when I was told the cancer was stage 2.

Fear started to take over with thoughts of the disease getting worse every time I went to the doctor.

I started to realize I had to get my fear in check, so I made the decision to focus on being positive and on my blessings.

It was the only way to get through it all.

After surgery and radiation, I couldn't use my left upper body like I had in the past and medication just made me feel like I was in a totally different body.

Movement with affirmations and transitioning to a plant based whole food diet including wheatgrass and sprouts helped me to gain confidence in what I considered a "new" body.

It really wasn't until the photoshoot I found beauty in the flaws.

This experience really has me in awe how beautiful the woman's body can be perfectly imperfect.

My best advice is to find what brings you joy and lean into it daily not only during a diagnosis but in everyday life.

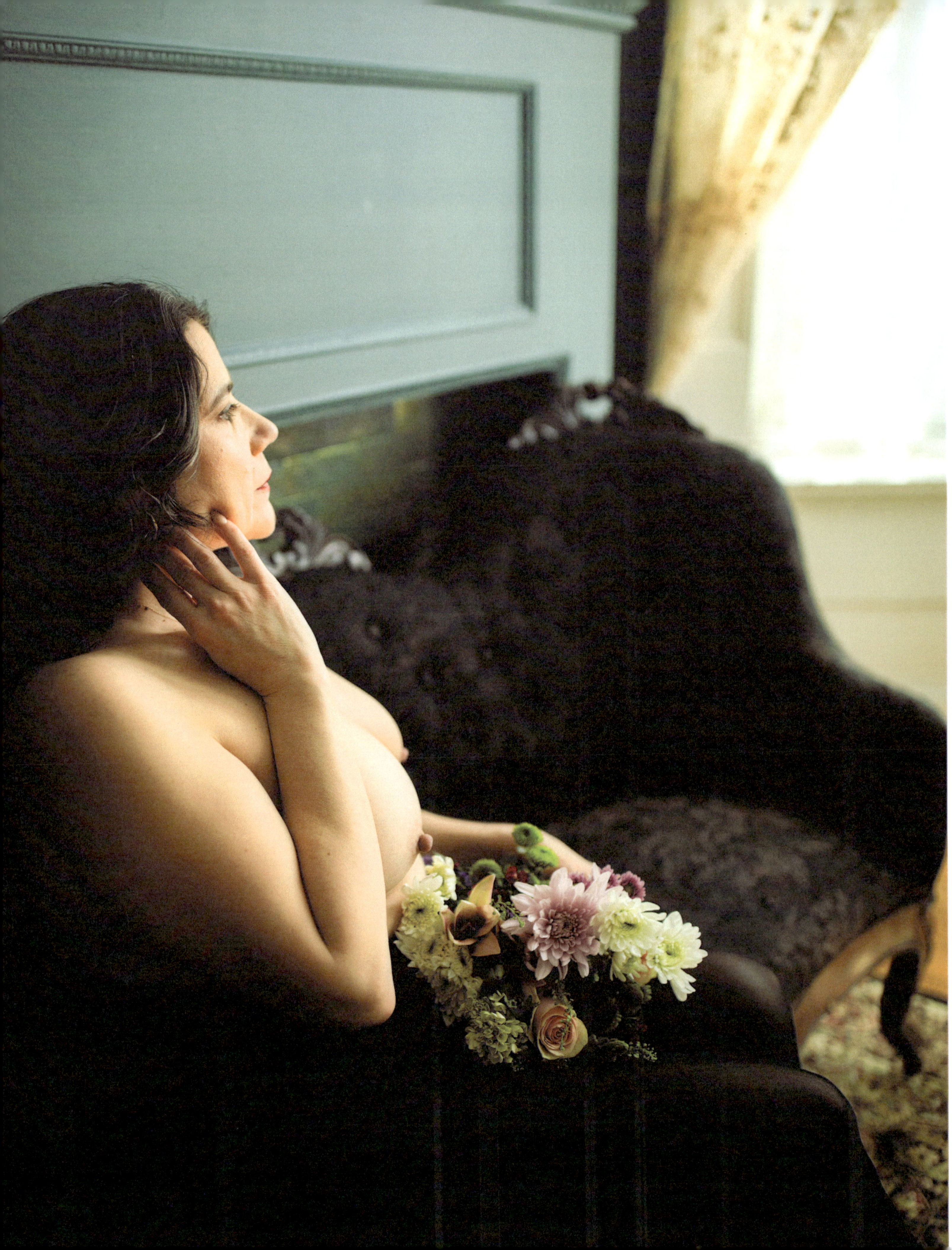

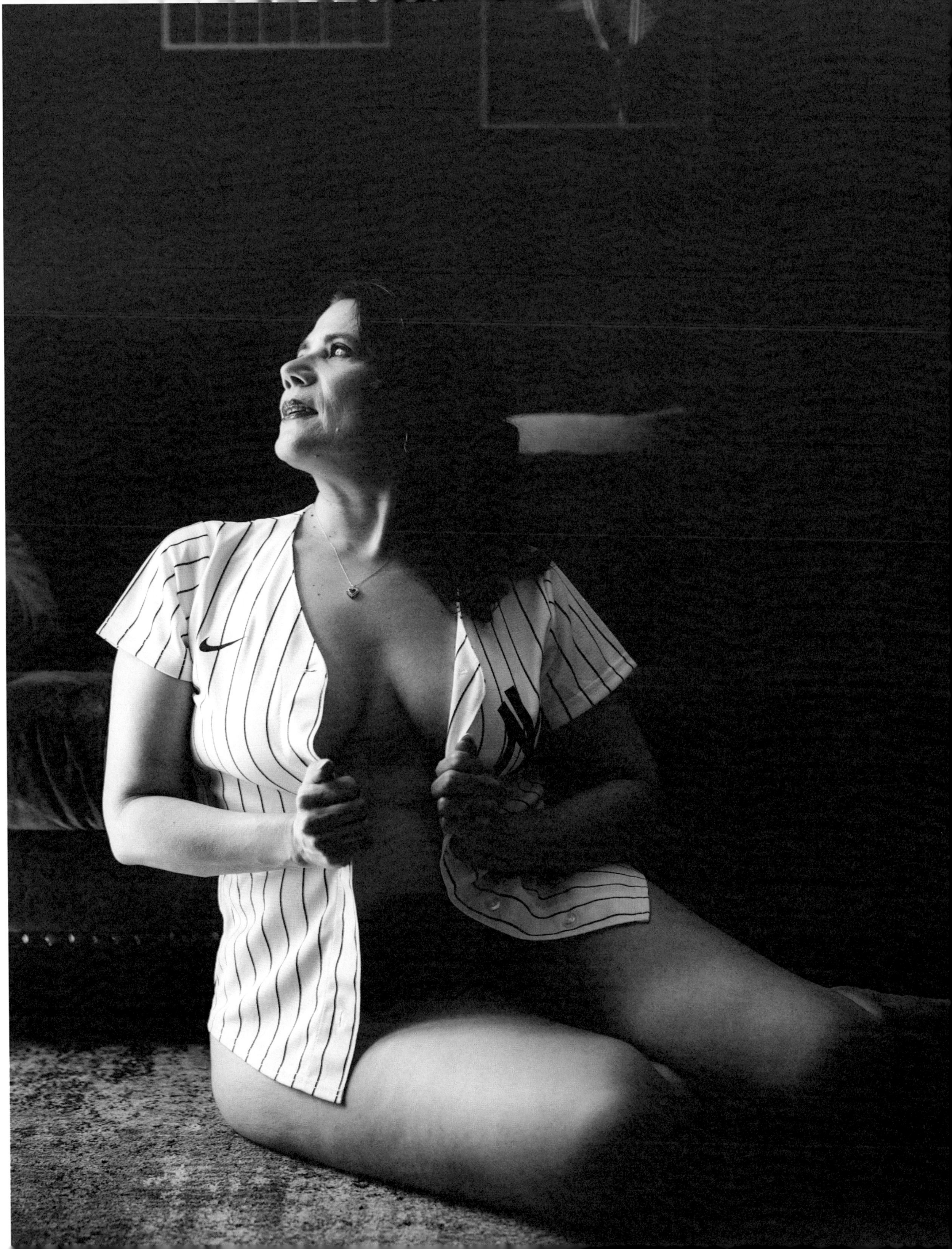

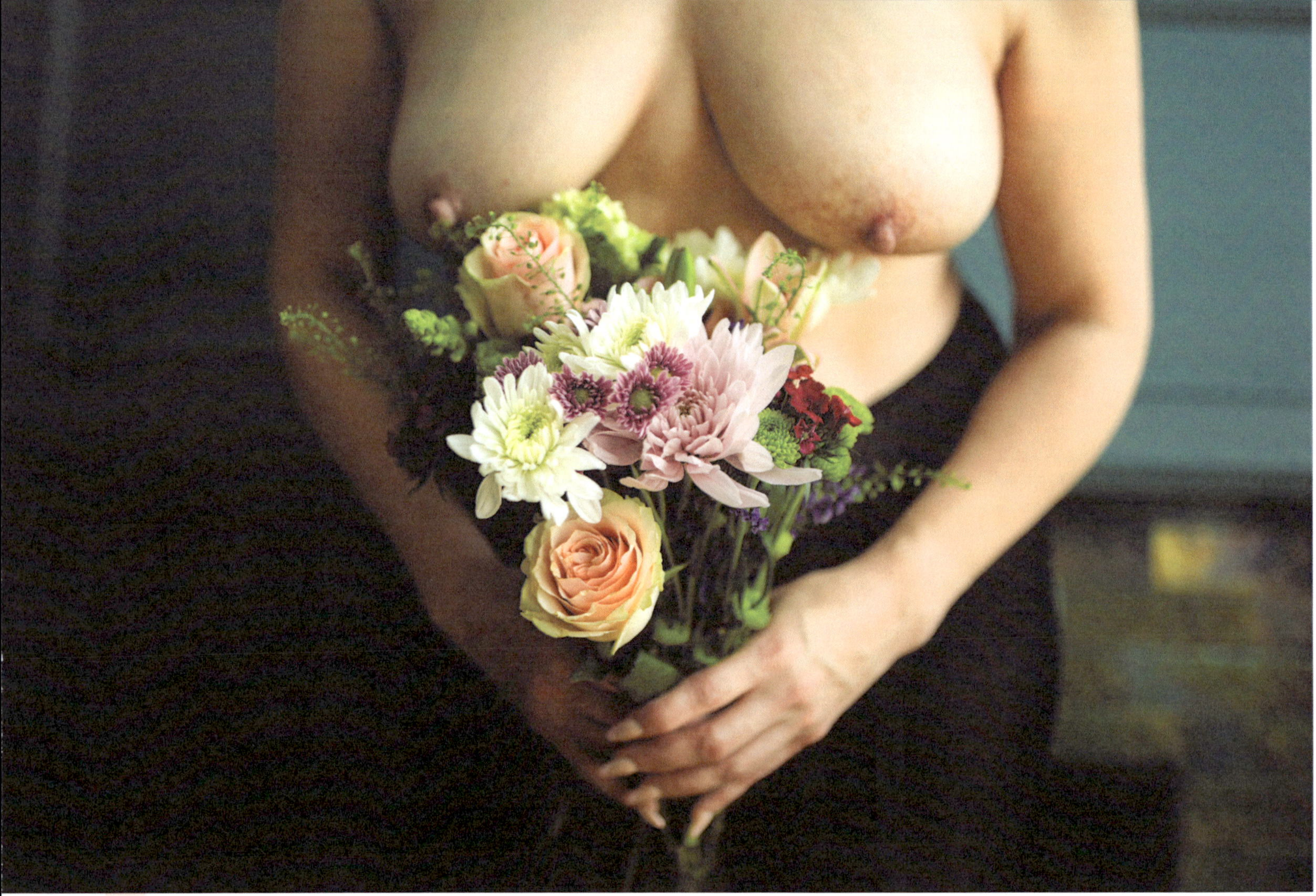

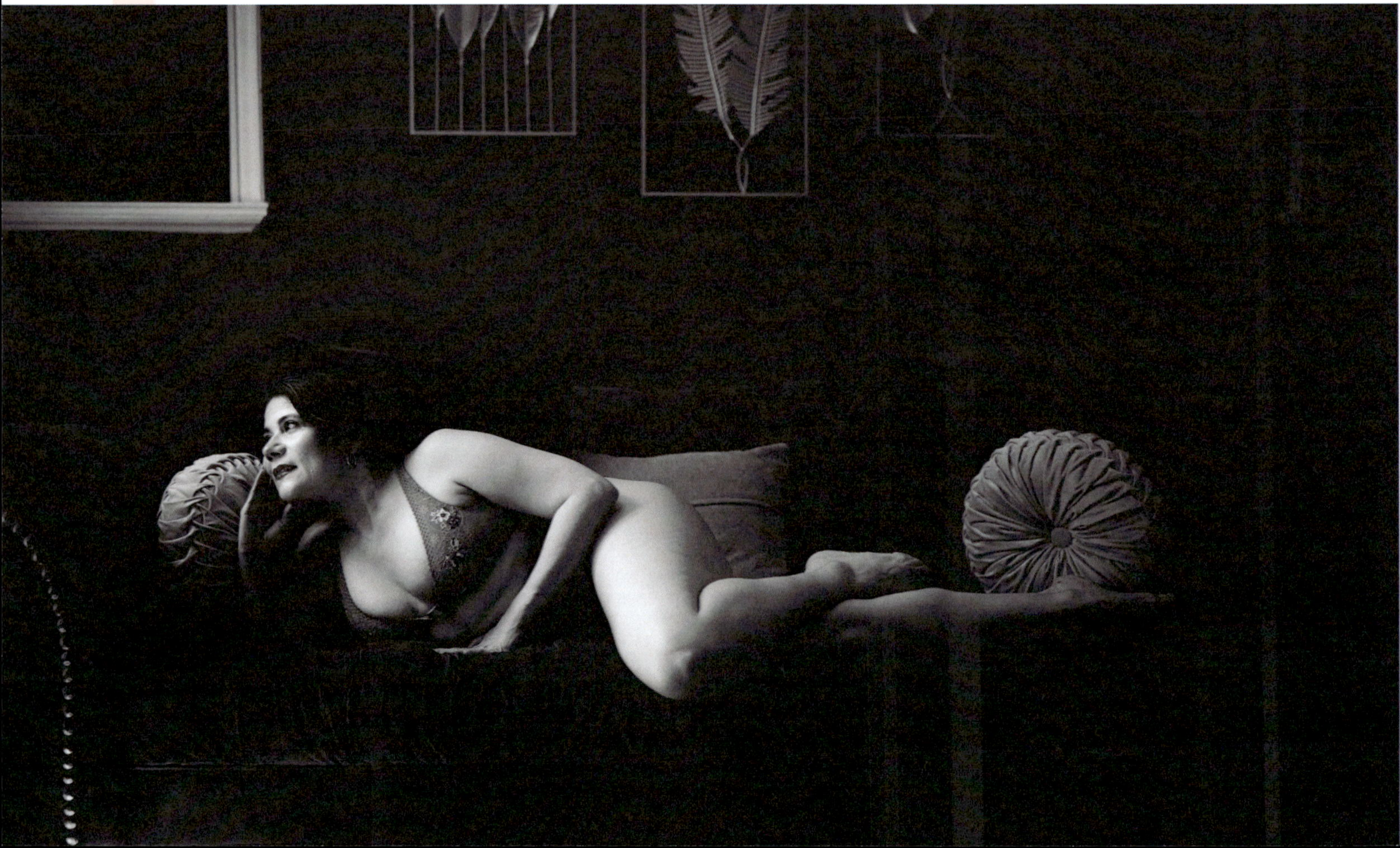

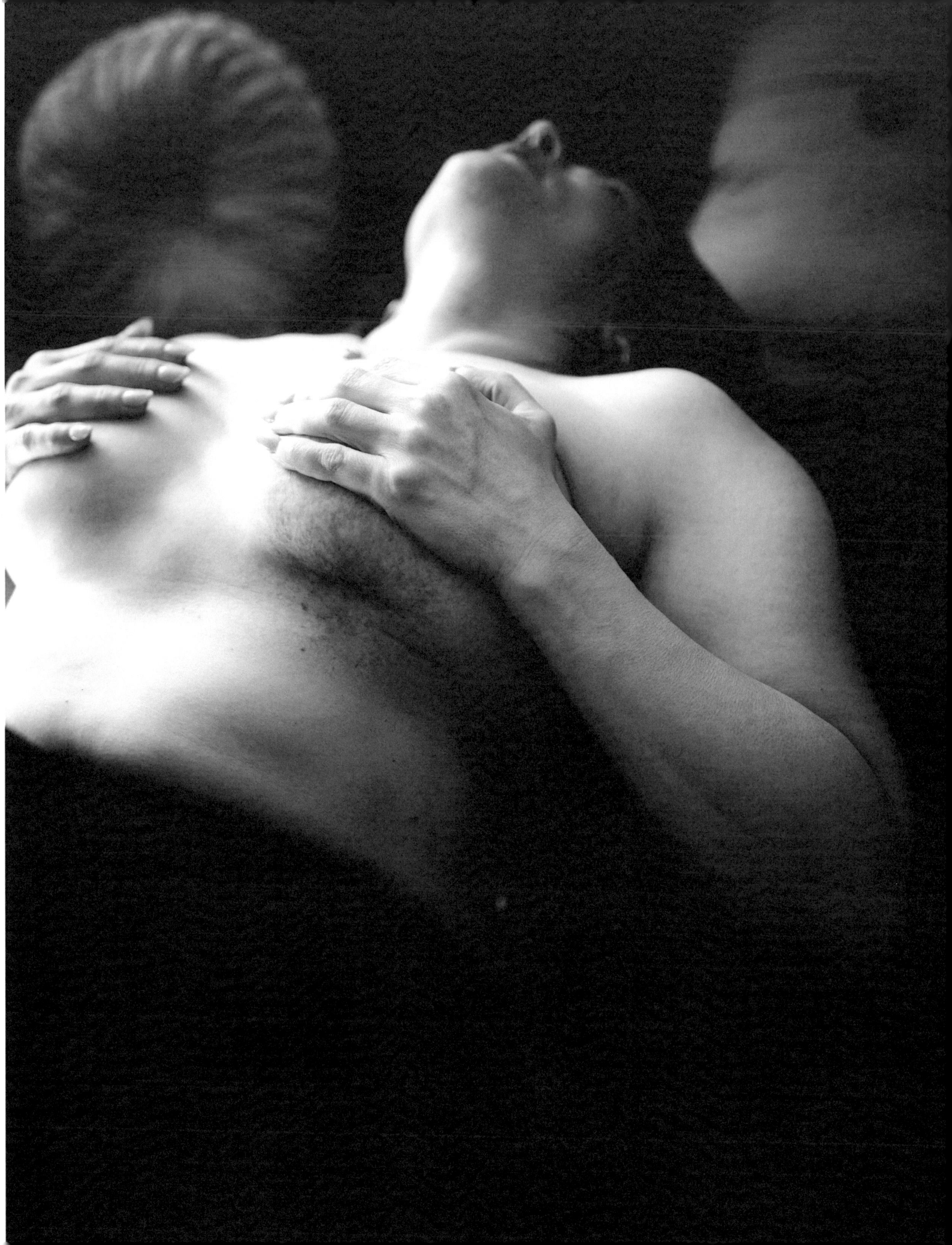

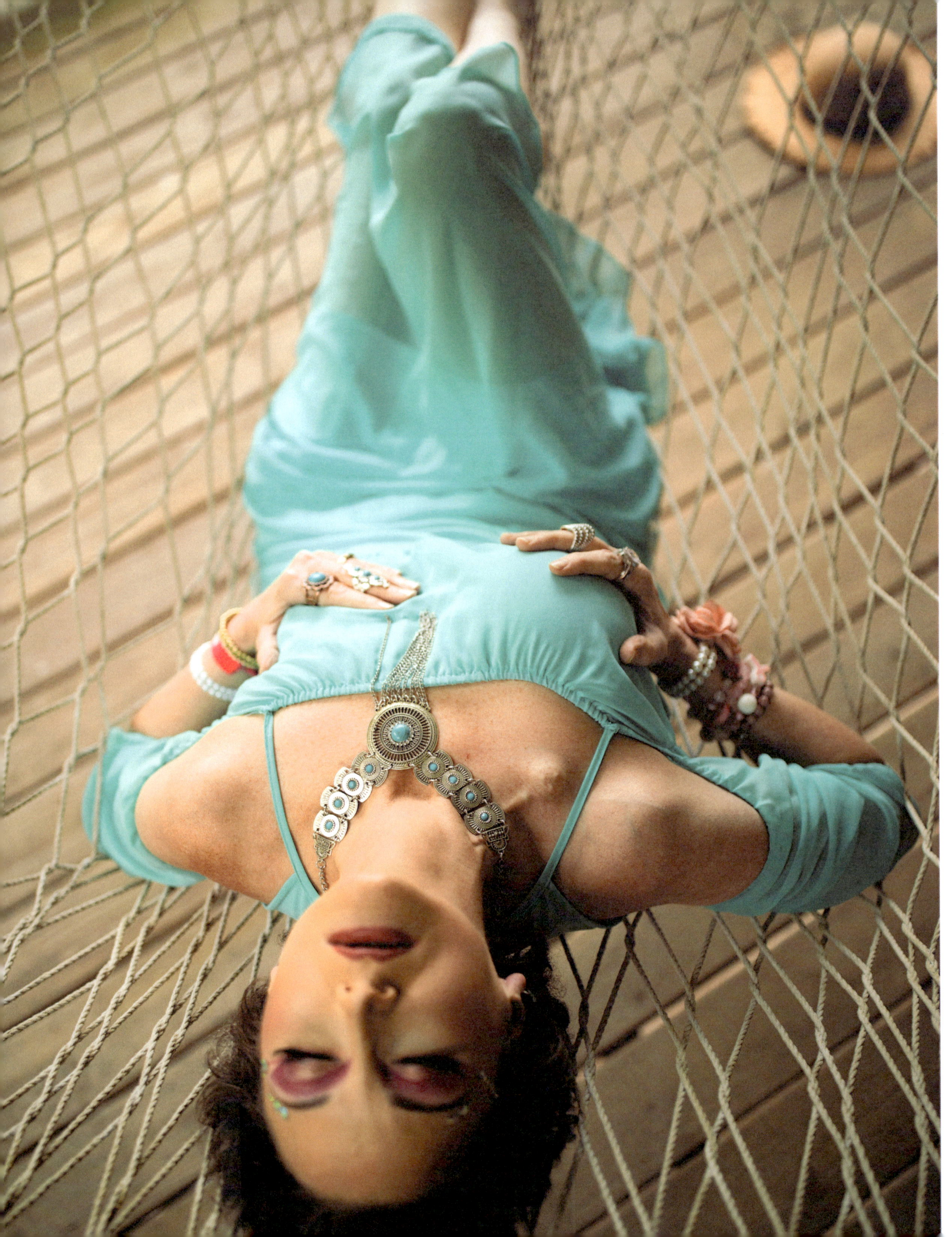

Diagnosis: *Breast Cancer*
Age Diagnosed: *48*
Treatments Received: *Chemo, radiation, cancer meds.*
Age at time of photographs: *48*
Stage at time of photographs: *Stage 2B*
Region: *North Carolina*
Social Media: *@windylougibson on FB*
@cancerqueencountrygirl on IG

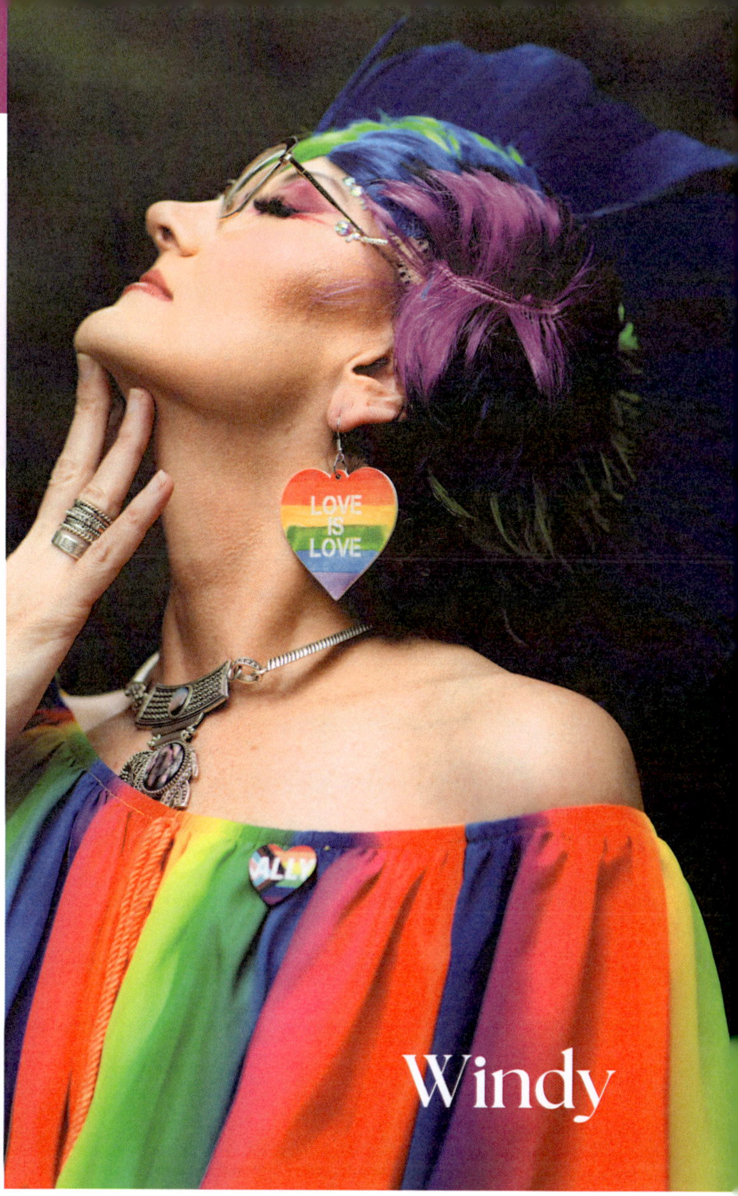

Windy

Alright Ladykins, put your big girl panties on, buckle up and get ready for the ride of life!

W.W.W. Windylou's Wackadoodle World.

Enter with caution.

My cancer journey started in 2022. I always wanted to be a part of a club but the Cancer club? No, no thank you ma'am but here I am!

I've never been comfortable or friends with my body. I got my reconstruction surgery in February.

2024, promptly broke my back 3 days before my 50th birthday, and lost my left breast again due to the back brace rubbing a hole in my breast and causing me to become sick. I became deeply depressed which was totally opposite of me when I was first diagnosed and during treatment.

I knew then that if I didn't get some therapy, I would tunnel myself into a dark twisting hole and may never come out. I found me a wonderful therapist at Bloom and balance, Miss Tony.

We are working on a journey of self-love, body love, and acceptance.

And if all else fails, child watch you some drag Queens. The Joy RuPaul's Drag Race brought for me during chemo rides to and fro to treatment is beyond measurable. And as Mama Ru always says " if you can't love yourself, how the hell you going to love somebody else?

Can I get a Amen?

In the name of Jesus, RuPaul, Dolly, and Elvis, may your journey give you the eyes of gratitude and joy 💕

As a child my precious mama told me to love thy neighbor to be like Jesus to be kind, considerate, and to stand up for the bullied. I took her advice that she instilled in me all throughout my life.

I stand for the people no matter race, gender, sexual orientation, etc. Love is Love as my earrings say! I will always fight for humanity.

I am a huge Ally for the LGBTQIA+ community.

The pledge of allegiance says under one nation under God indivisible, Liberty and justice for ALL!!!

If your family has cashed you out, I offer free Mom hugs, you can come join the House of WinDiva Jolean Von Sugarbaker (that's my drag queen name when I make it big.) .

I'm sending love, light and prayers to the world and everyone in it!

Peace out Kitty Girls from Good ole North Carolina!

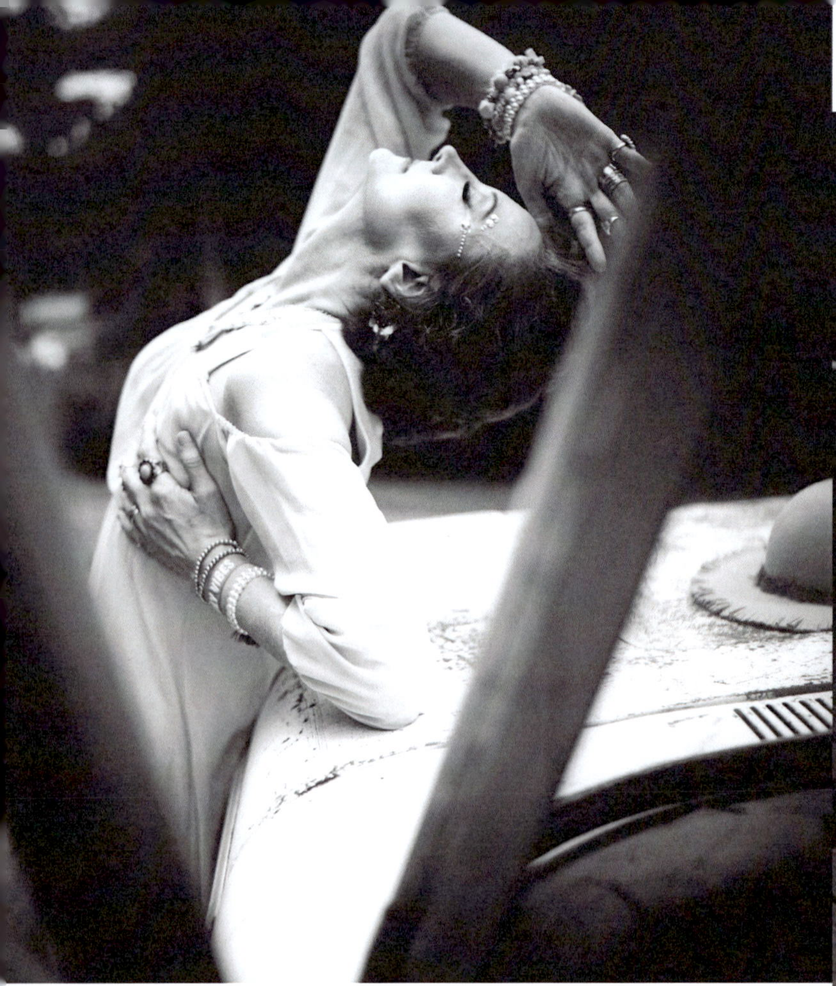

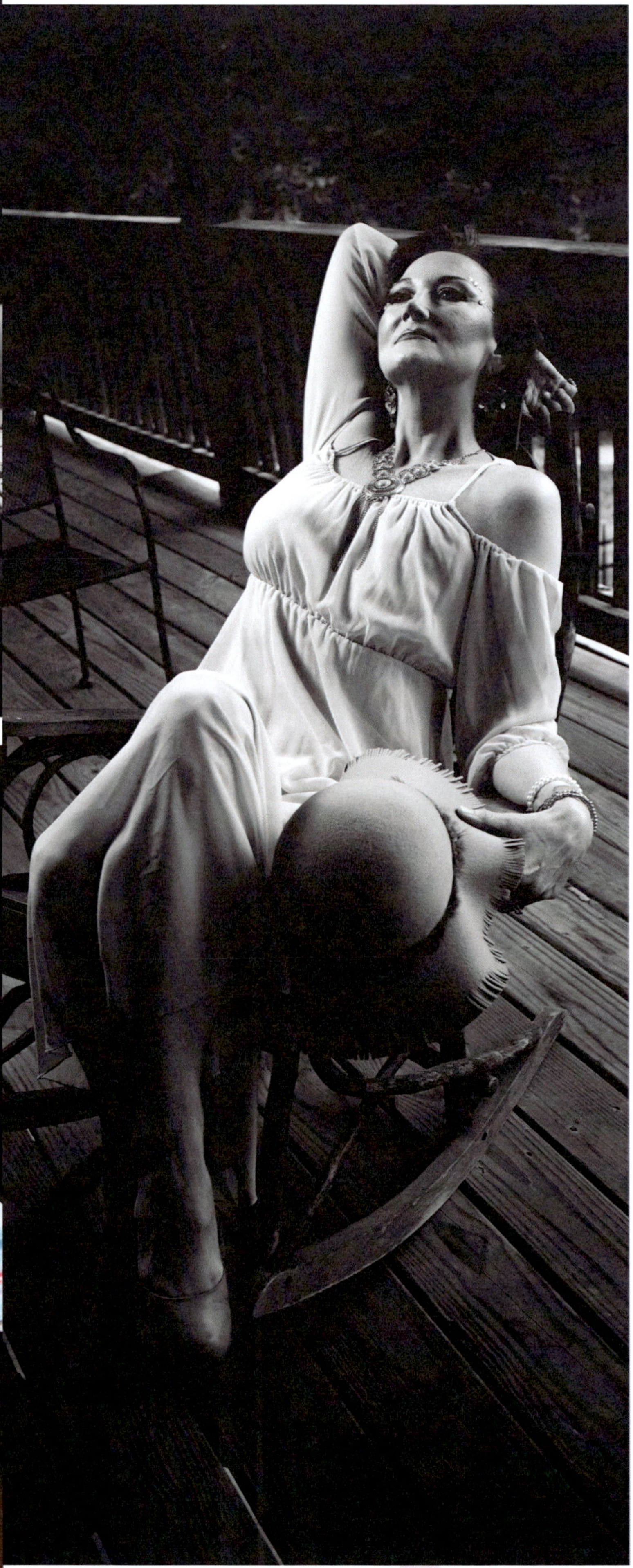

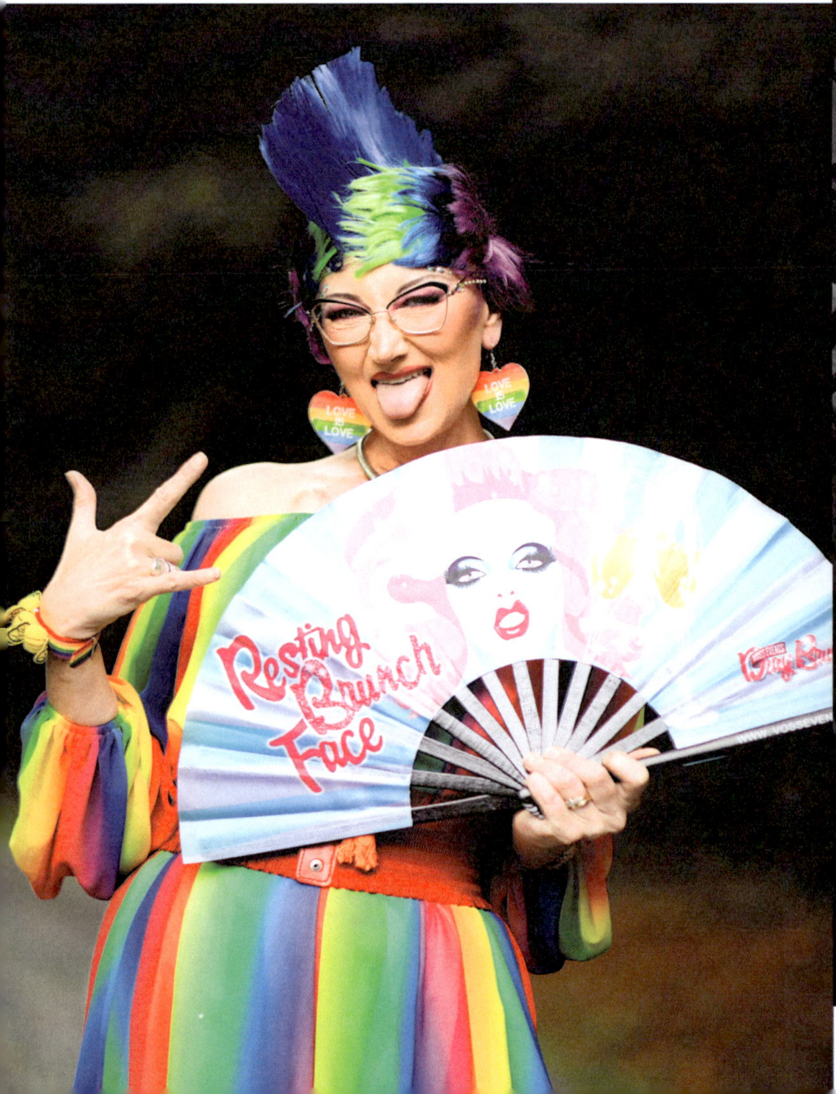
Resting Brunch Face

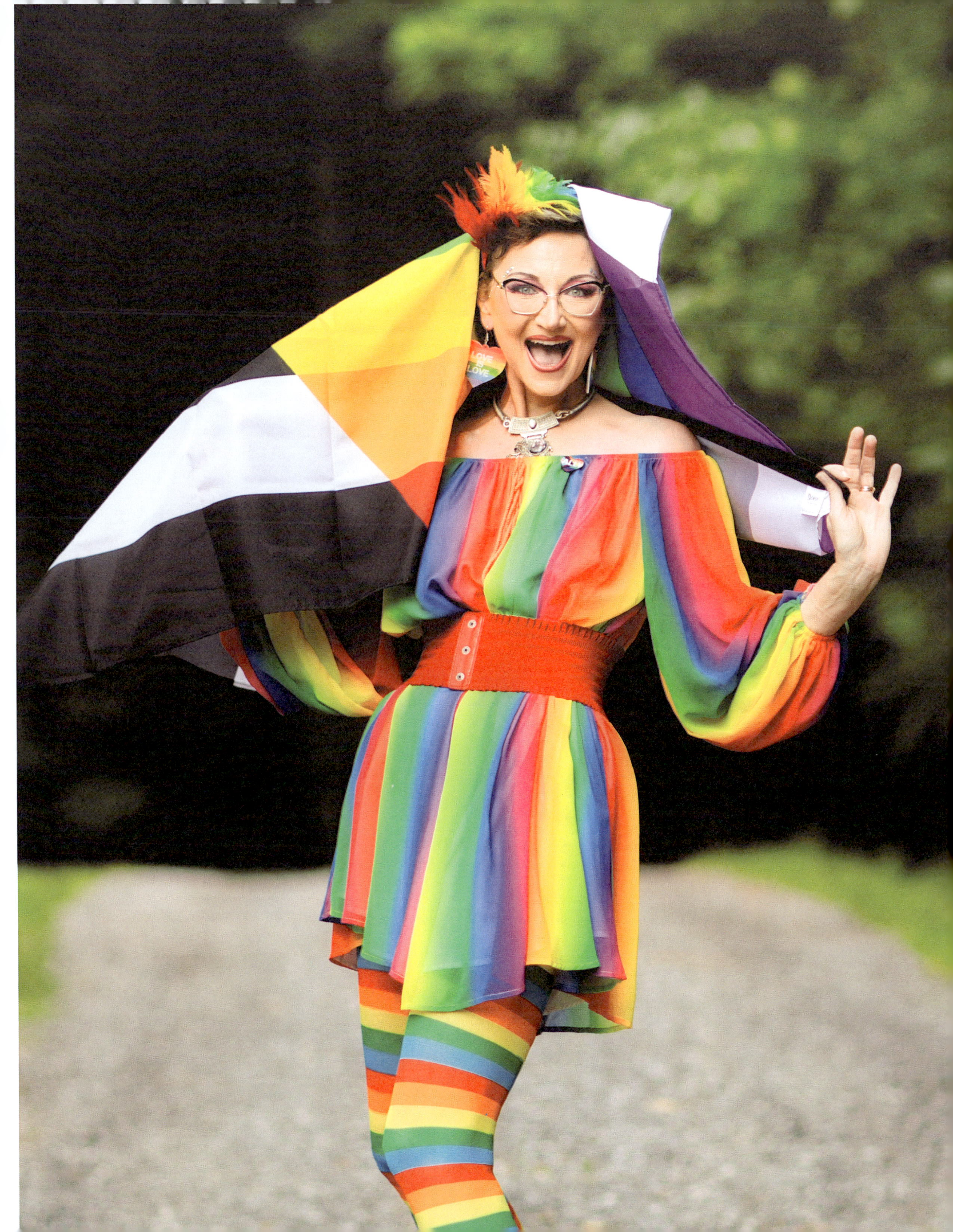
LOVE
LOVE

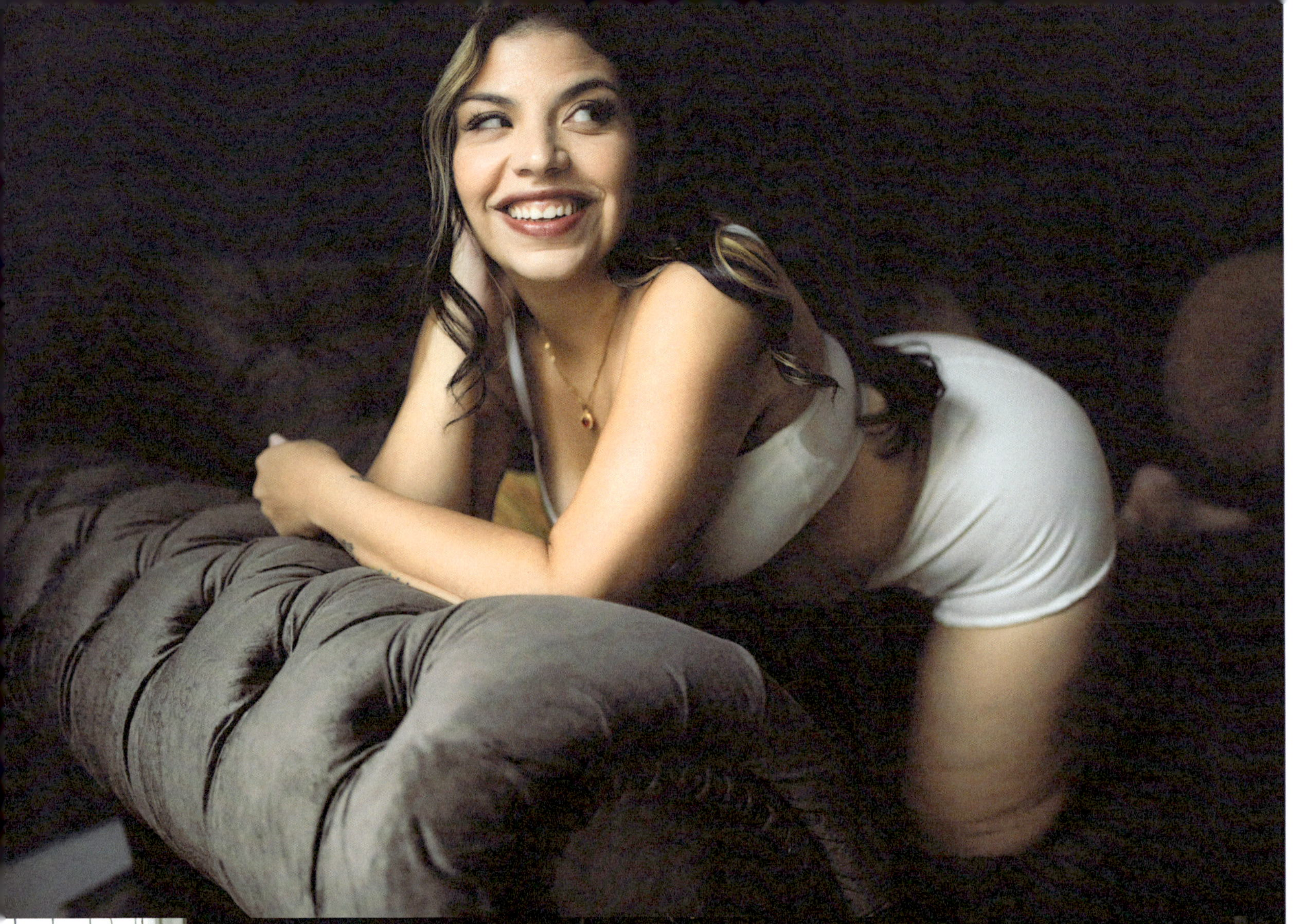

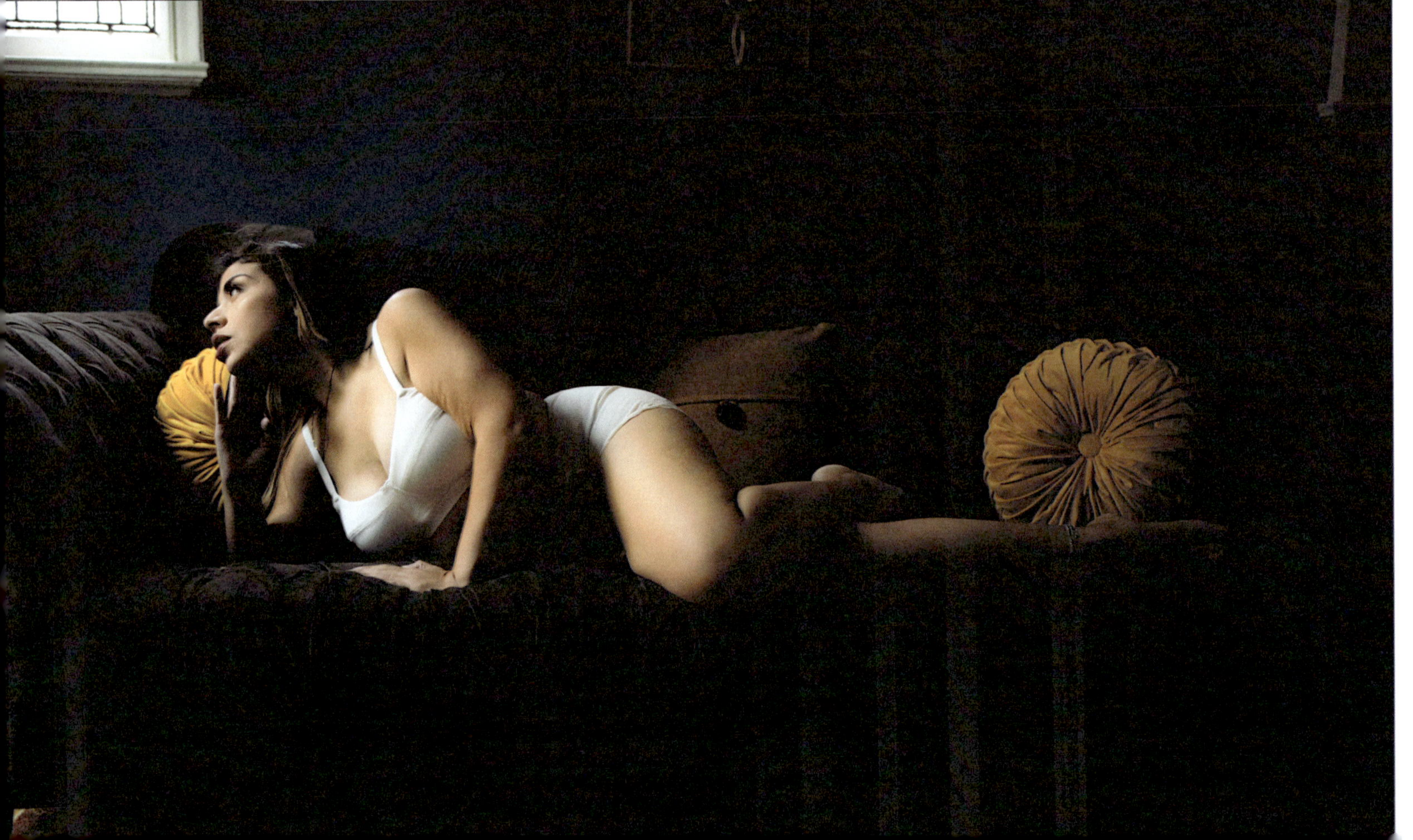

Diagnosis: *Genetics: BRCA2+ Tumor: Stage 2b Invasive Ductal Carcinoma ER & PR+, HER2-*
Age Diagnosed: *31*
Treatments Received: *Double Mastectomy,*
15 rounds of chemotherapy (AC+T),
25 rounds of radiation,
By salpingectomy & ovary removal,
TRAM flap recon surgery,
currently on hormone therapy
Age at time of photographs: *35*
Stage at time of photographs: *Post Treatment - NED*
Region: *Massachusetts*
Social Media: *@breastcancer_chingona*

Yahira

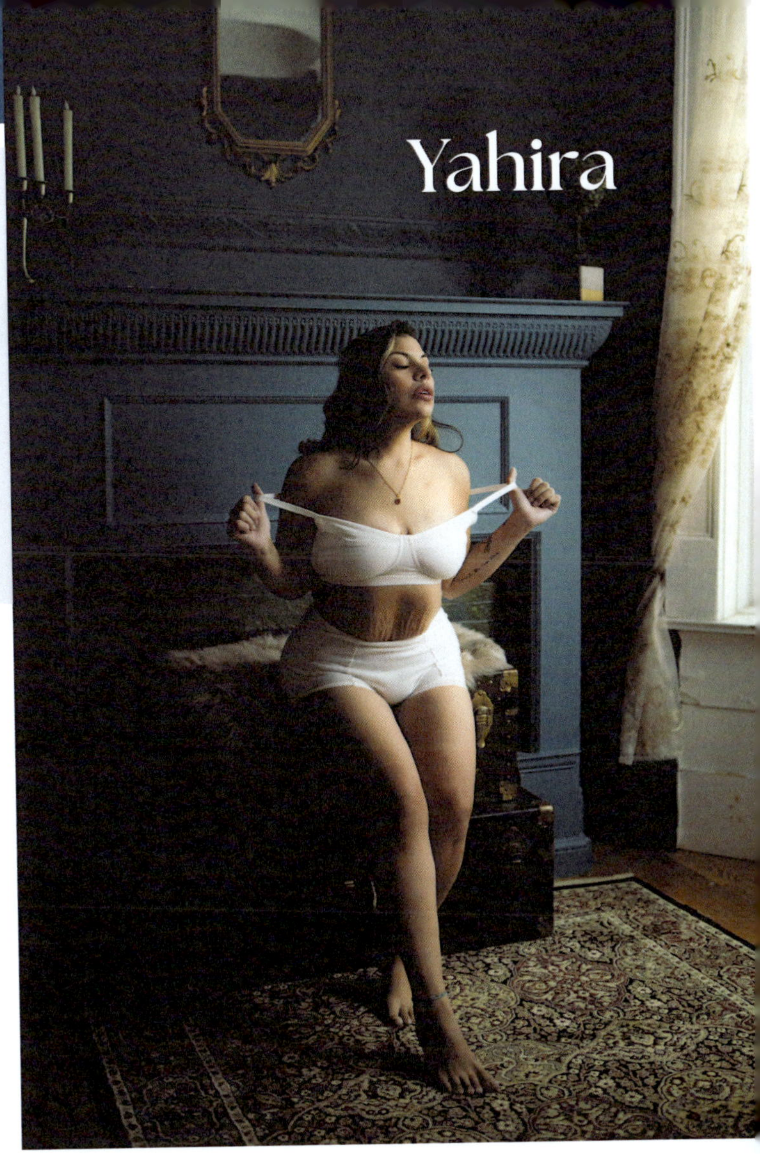

I often reflect on the various bodies I've inhabited throughout my life.

It's intriguing because I haven't always appreciated every version of myself. However, each transformation has narrated my life's journey and challenges. Growing up, I perceived myself as the "fat girl," and looking back at old photos, I recognized that my self-image was distorted by the comments of others.

Eventually, I learned to embrace my body and cultivate self-love through tools like fashion and photography. Then came motherhood, and with it, new changes to my body. I had to accept what this phase meant for me physically.

Without those early experiences and the lessons I learned about self-acceptance, I could have faced significant struggles when I was diagnosed with breast cancer.

I was advised to lose over 50 pounds to qualify for fat grafting breast reconstruction. Despite my efforts, losing the weight proved to be a challenge, leading me to choose bypass surgery. Following the surgery, I successfully lost a total of 100 pounds, marking another significant transformation in my body. Each physical transformation presents a mental hurdle that requires attention – and it can be incredibly draining.

Capture as many photos of your whole experience. Even if you are not fond of what you see in the mirror, and/or choose not to share them with anyone else. You will be surprised how much your body transforms, and what it can endure. Reflecting on various stages of my time has allowed me to appreciate everything my body has been through and its capabilities. Each scar tells a story, and that is, in itself, incredibly powerful.

Find your people. Seek out individuals who genuinely support you, who don't contribute to your stress, and if you can - find folks who truly understand your struggle. Finding a community was a game changer for me. It helped me feel less alone, and was a great resource for me when I felt defeated.

People like to compare cancer to a battle. I do not like seeing it that way - because no one "loses" the battle of cancer. You don't need to be constantly "fighting for your life", or "showing face". Rest as much as possible, stay hydrated, and let yourself ride out your emotions.

Take it one day at a time, one step at a time - and focus on small joys, and practicing gratitude when navigating through hard moments.

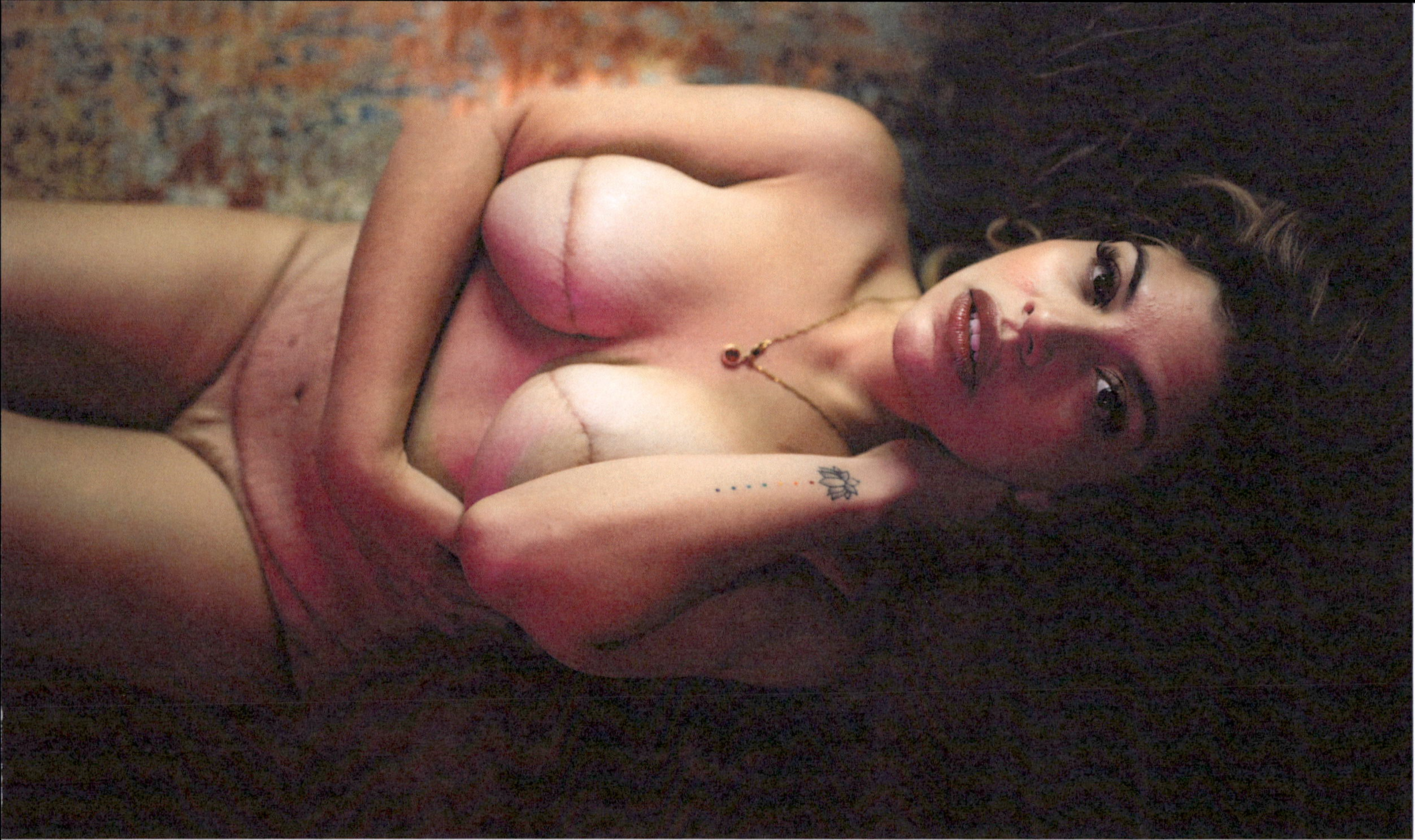

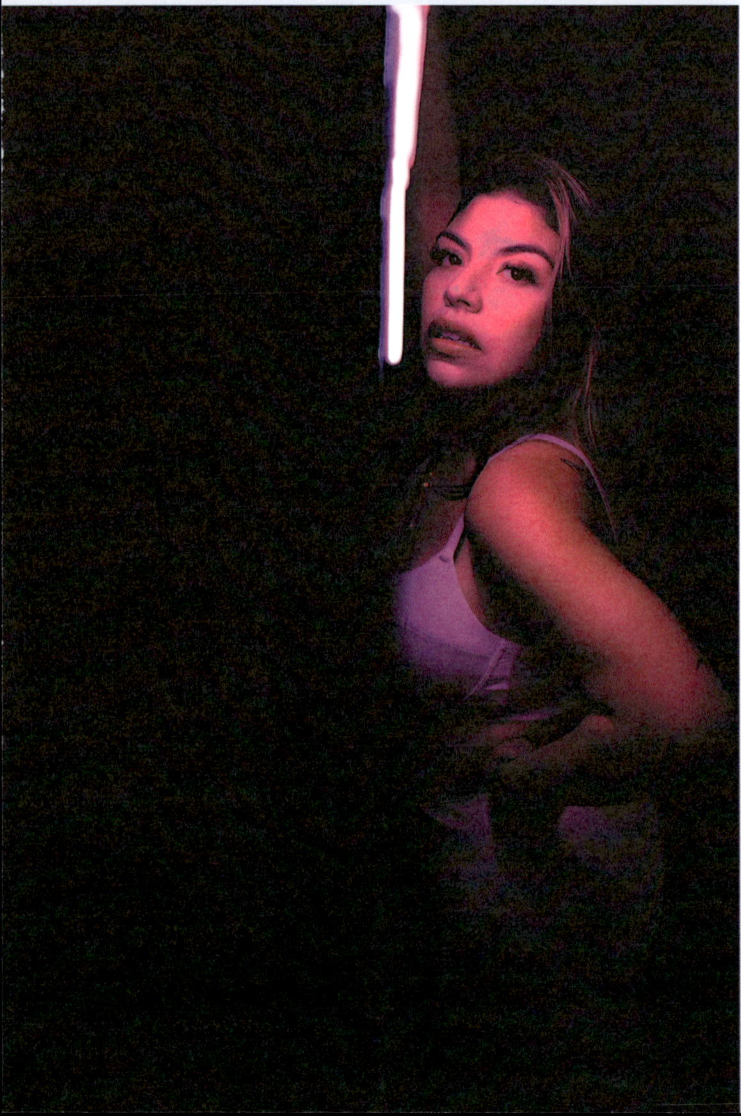

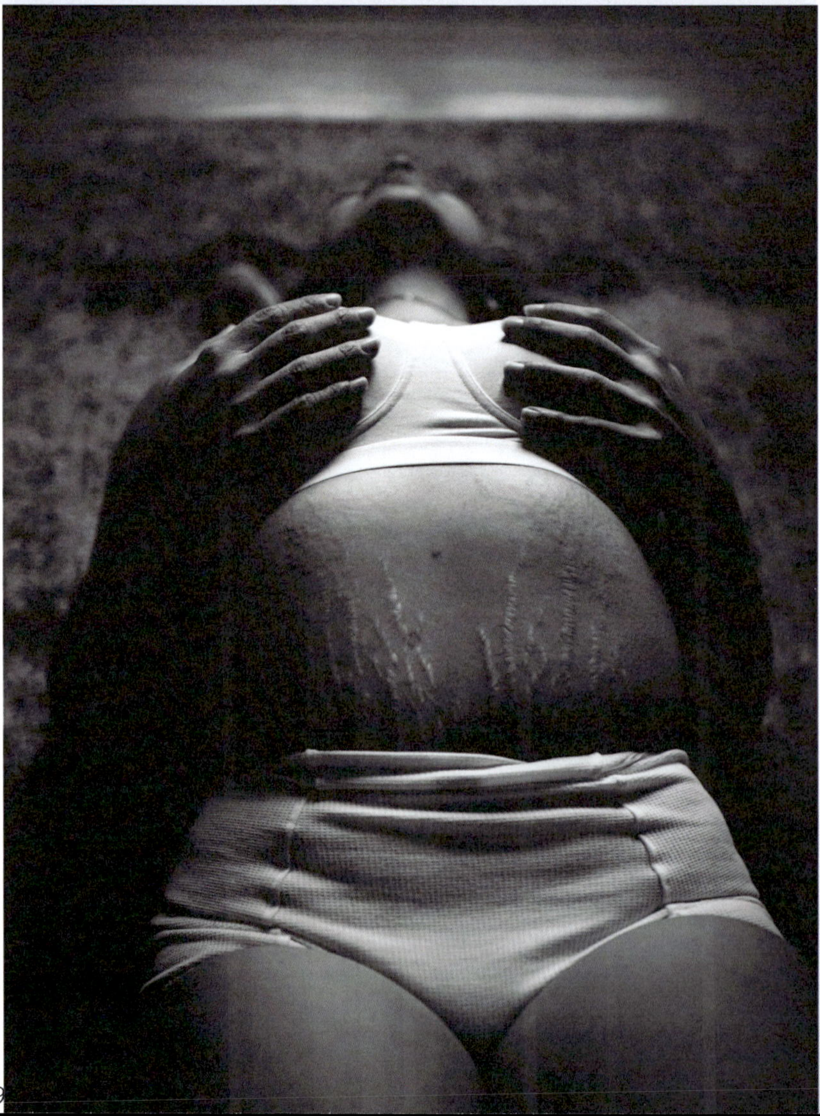

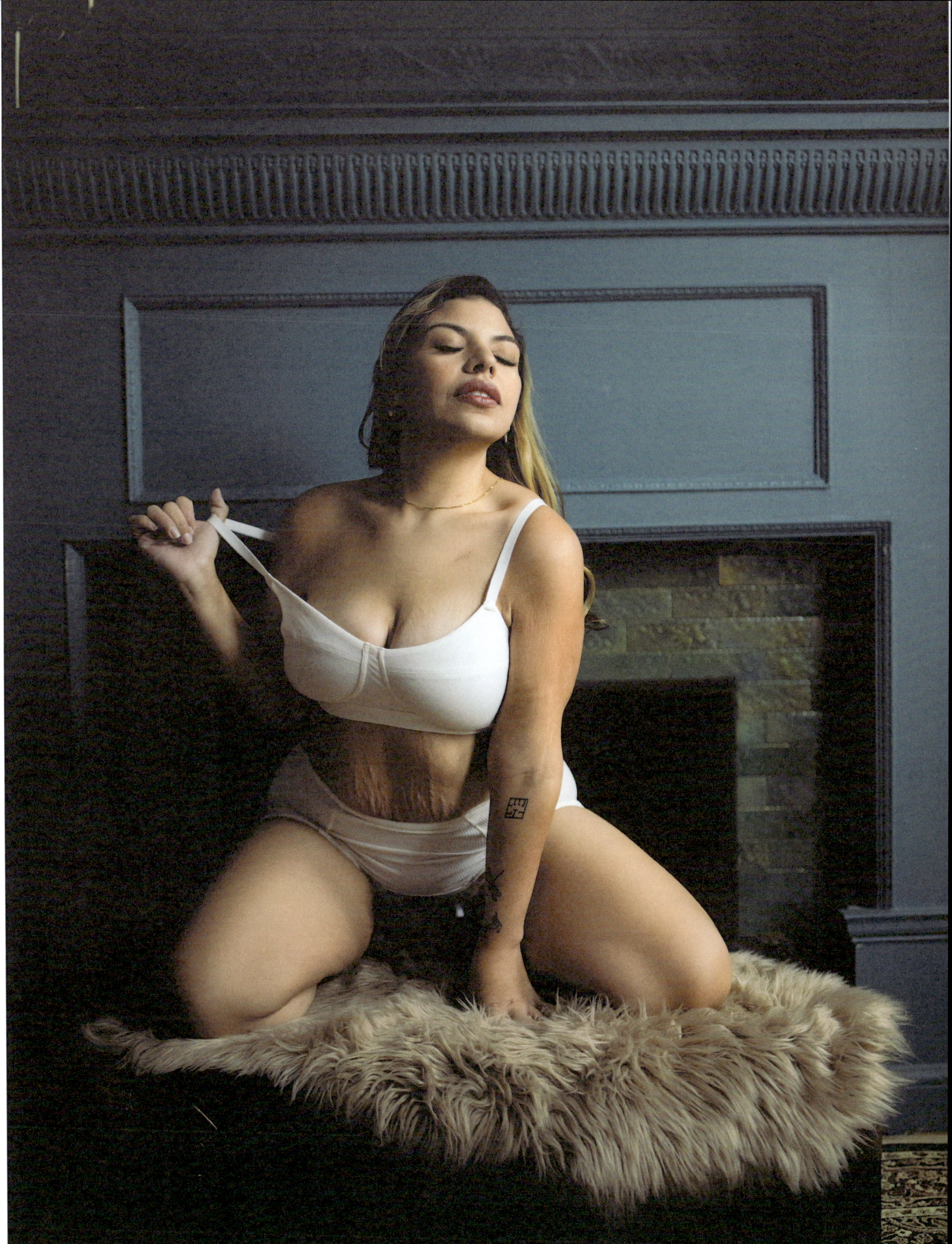

AESTHETIC FLAT CLOSURE

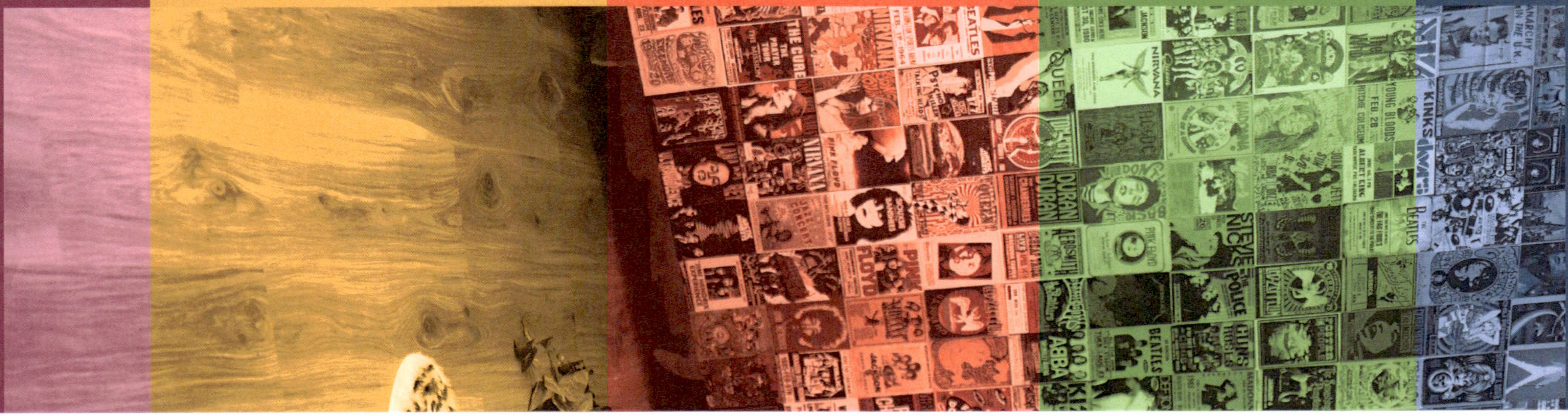

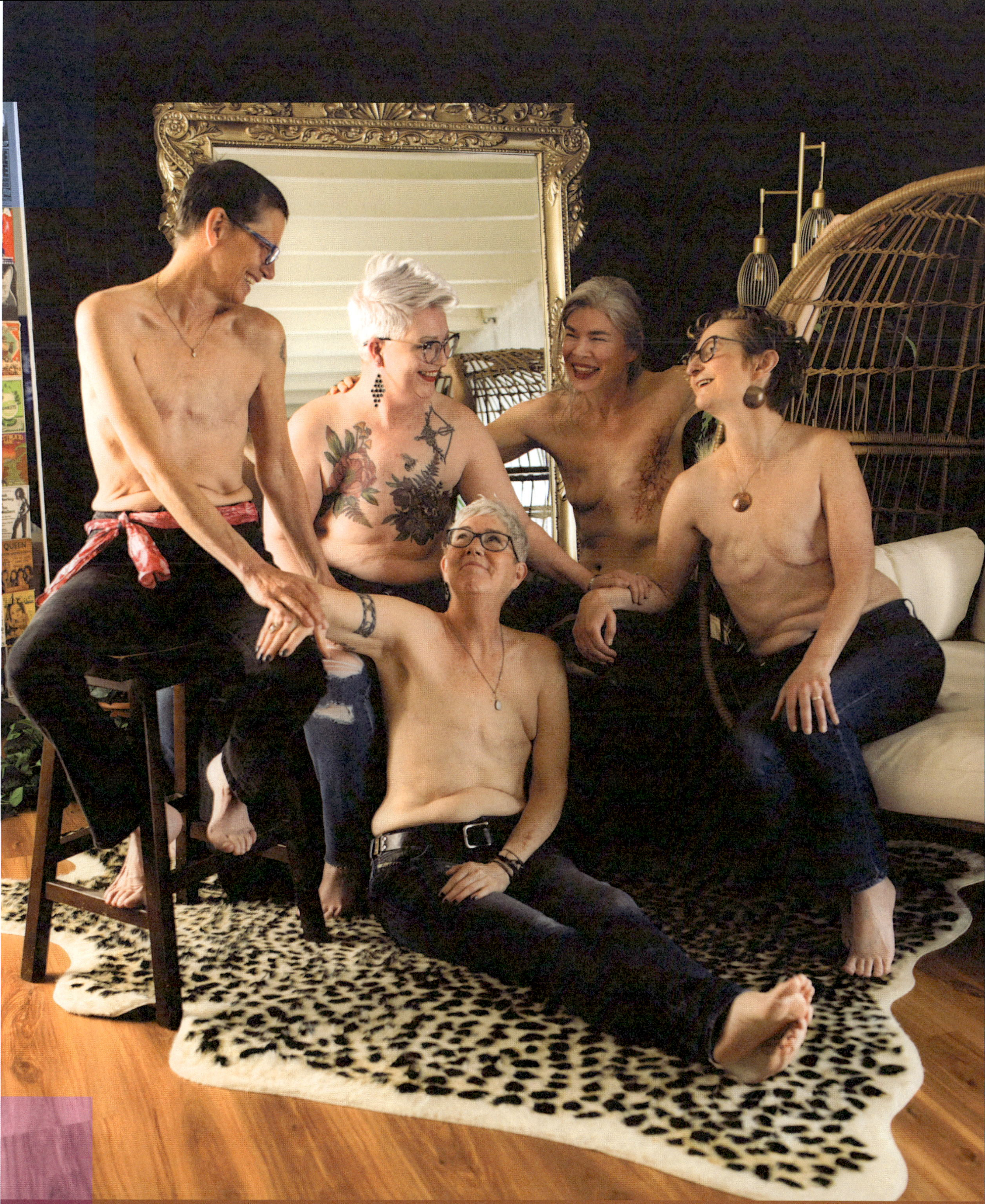
QUEEN

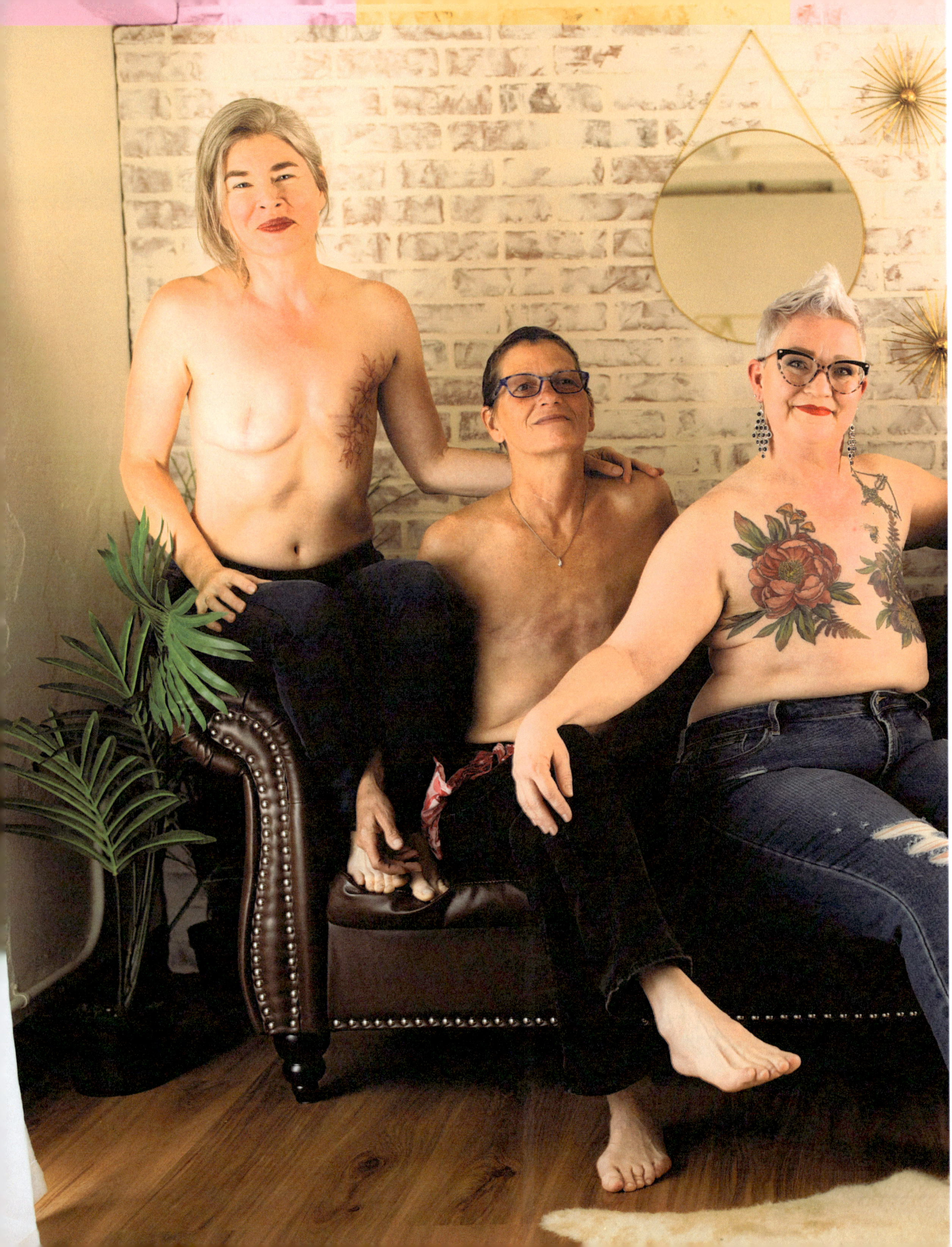

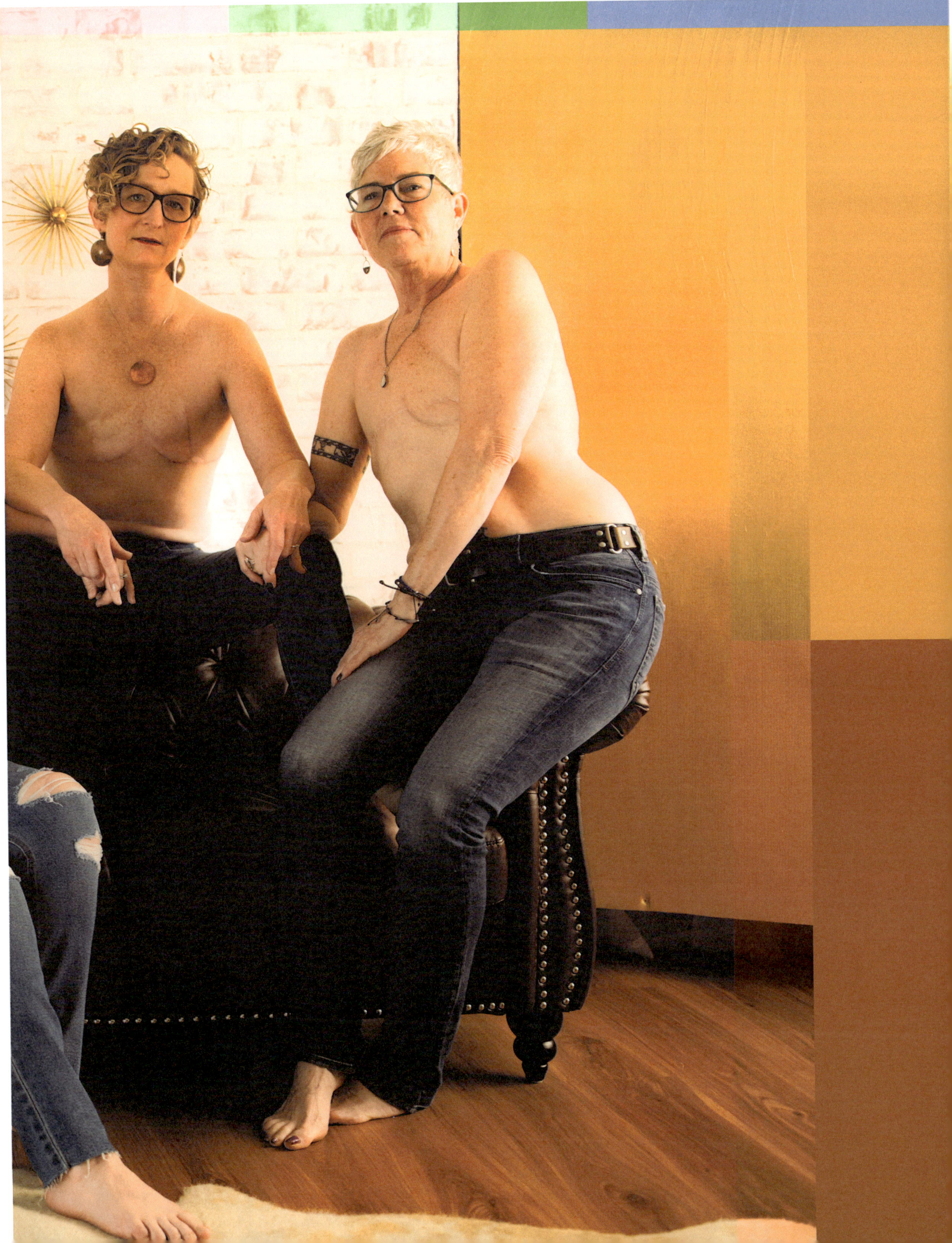

Kira

Diagnosis: *Hormone positive, HER2 negative Invasive mammary carcinoma with ductal and lobular features, grade 2. Two years later I had a positive lymph node.*
Age Diagnosed: *45*
Treatments Received: *First I just had a mastectomy then started hormone blockers. Two years later I was diagnosed again with a positive lymph node. I then did TC chemo, a lymph node dissection, a hysterectomy and then radiation. That was followed by two years of Verzenio and 5-10 years of an AI.*
Age at time of photographs: *49*
Stage at time of photographs: *Cancer free!*
Region: *Northwest, Oregon*

Going through cancer has shown me how truly fortunate I am.

When faced with very difficult decisions and exhausting treatments, I was surrounded by love, support and amazing medical teams.

I knew that my body would have a hard time accepting any type of implants.

I also knew that my relationship with the breasts I had would be forever changed. When I heard about aesthetic flat closure, it just made sense to me.

I have not regretted this decision a single day.

I am proud of my choices and proud of my body.

To see the actions of a true village of support has renewed our outlook on humanity. It is hard to live in this world sometimes.

But seeing how people have come together to support our family has restored that faith in humanity.

Kathleen

Diagnosis: *Lobular Breast Cancer*
Age Diagnosed: *49*
Treatments Received: *Surgery*
Age at time of photographs: *51*
Stage at time of photographs: *No evidence of disease*
Region: *Northwest*
Social Media: *abreastcancerdiary.substack.com*

Breast cancer helped me to conquer some of my body-history that I didn't want to address or even face.

I felt a much more urgent need to love my body after my mastectomies.

My ability to reclaim confidence and pride in my body after my mastectomies was a surprise to me.

The flat community has a levity about it-- not glossing over our losses, but seeing the community itself as a way to "belong" to a new definition of beauty, and to adopt a new set of beliefs that meet us each time we look in the mirror.

My biggest hurdle after breast cancer was loneliness.

It took me six months to find community of friends and a support group that I could fully let my feelings out with.

Now, after seeking and finding a solid group of friends, I have the right level of support and self expression.

I have deep needs in the area of self disclosure, self knowledge and self expression, and once I found others who fit the same description, I was no longer adrift socially.

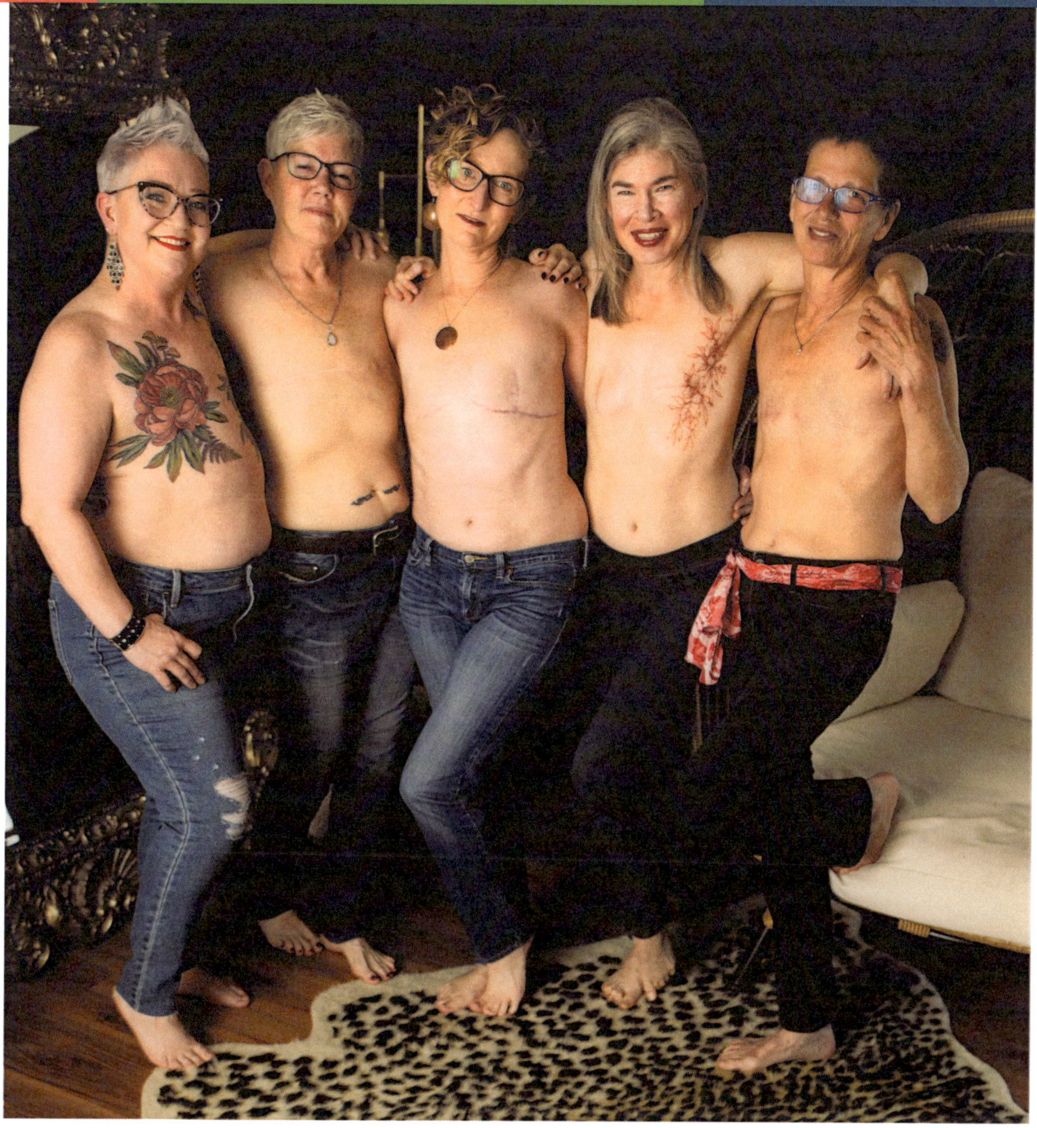

Tracy

Diagnosis: Dcis ductal breast cancer.
Age Diagnosed: 57
Treatments Received: AFC surgery, chemotherapy.
Age at time of photographs: 59
Stage at time of photographs: Remission
Region: Oregon

Wendy

Diagnosis: Breast cancer
Age Diagnosed: 58
Treatments Received: Double mastectomy w/ aromatase inhibitors.
Age at time of photographs: 59
Stage at time of photographs: Stage 2
Region: PNW / Oregon
Social Media: @wendy.murray.5492

Danyel

Diagnosis: Originally diagnosed in 2022 with Triple Negative Breast Cancer. In 2024 became metastatic to my lungs, liver and brain.
Age Diagnosed: 47
Treatments Received: 4 rounds Taxotere, double mastectomy, 17 rounds of Taxol, 7 rounds of Trodelvy.
Age at time of photographs: 49
Stage at time of photographs: Completed and considered NED
Region: Oregon
Social Media: @warriorwomenportraits

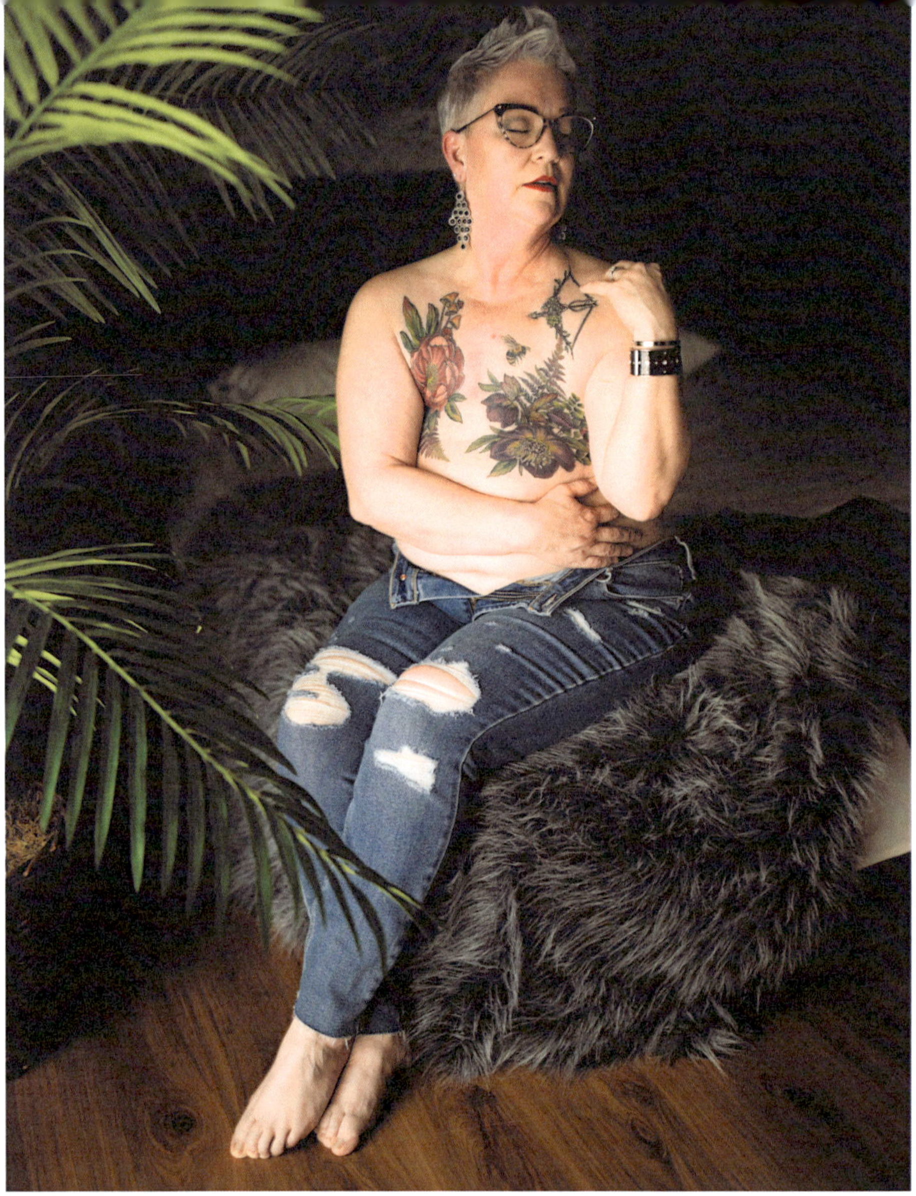

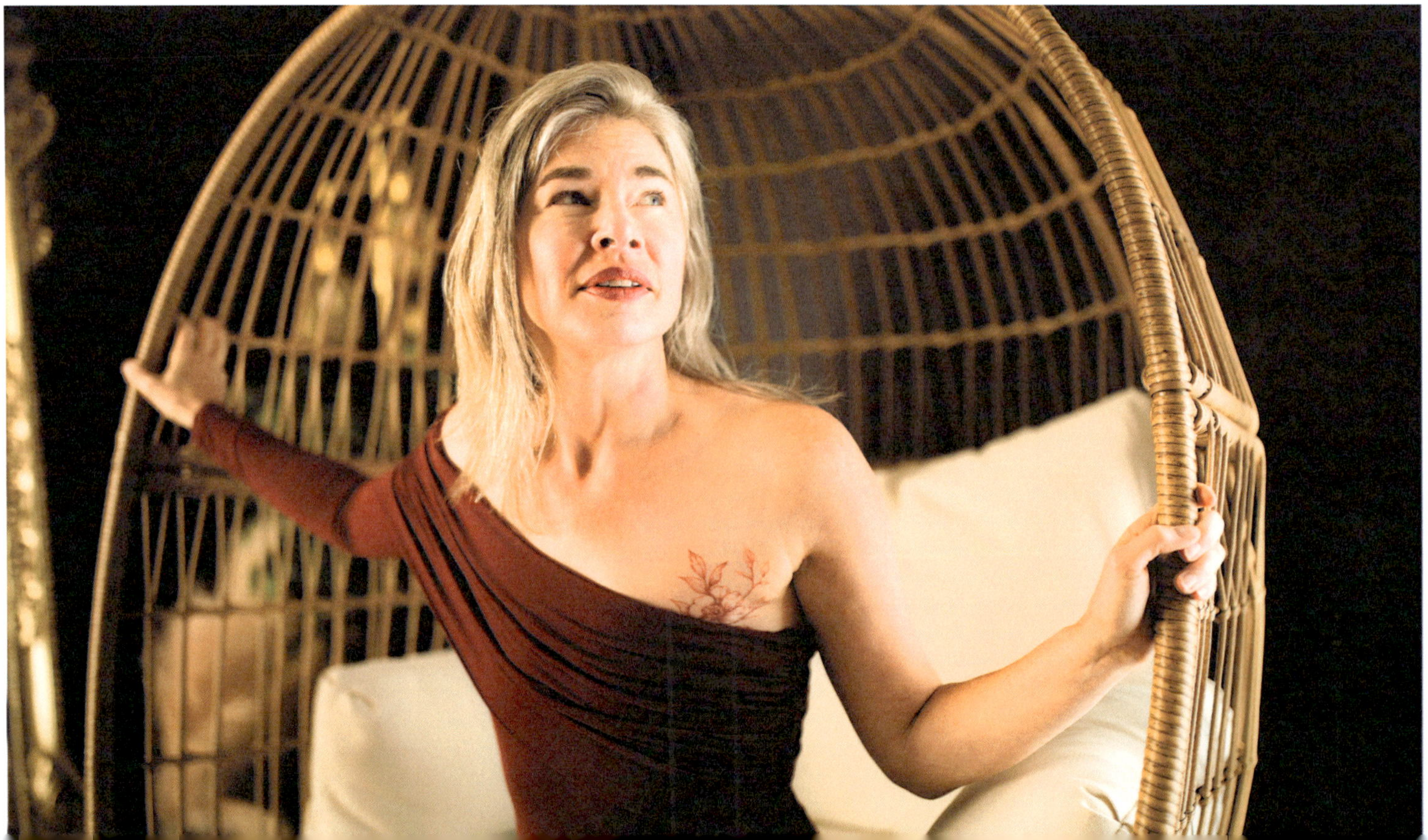

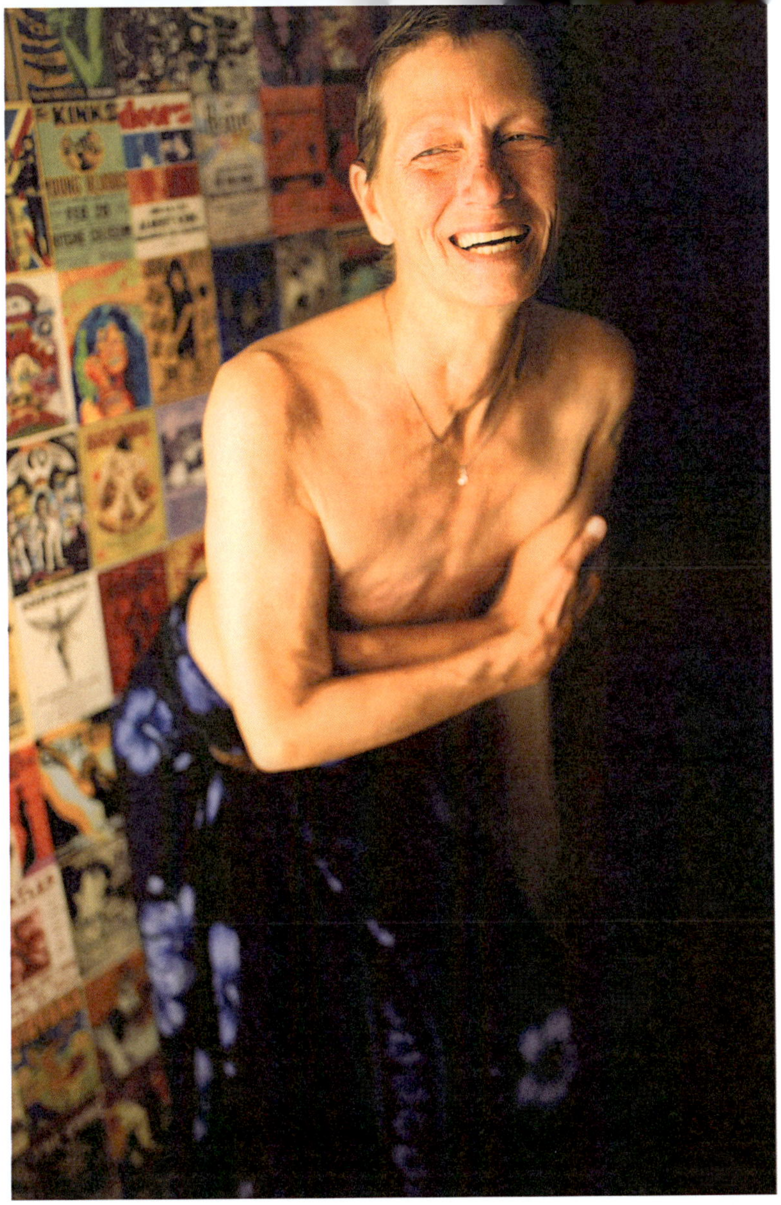
KINKS
doors

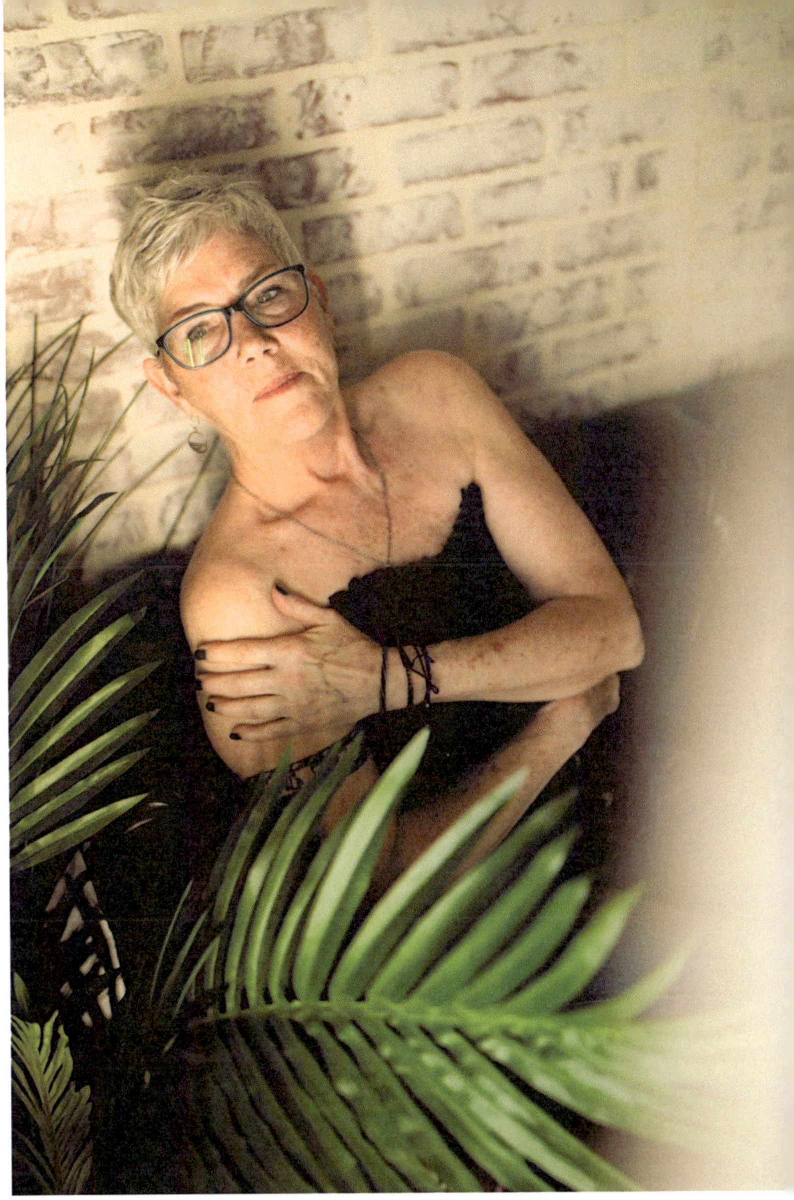

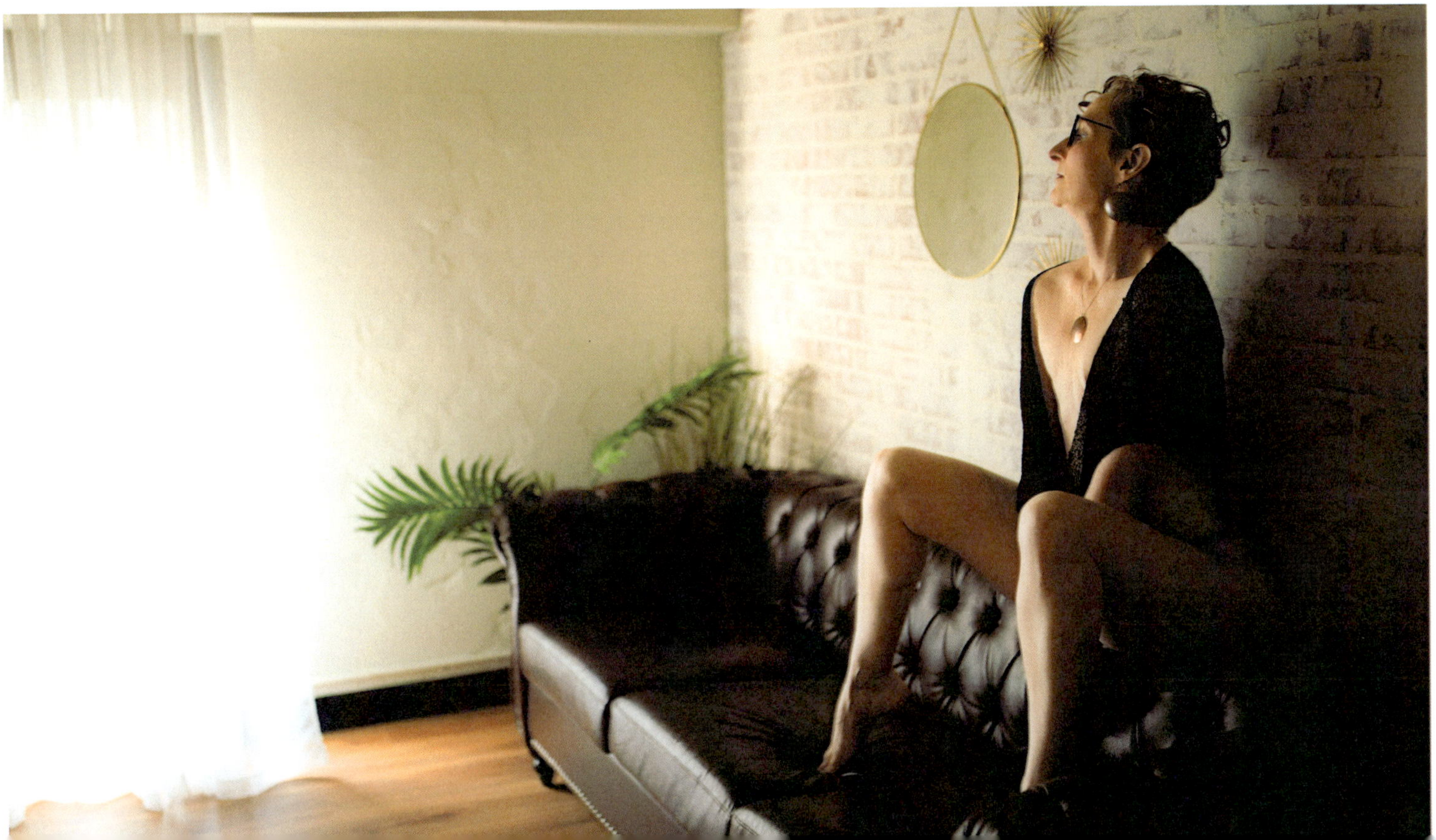

About the Project & Non-Profit

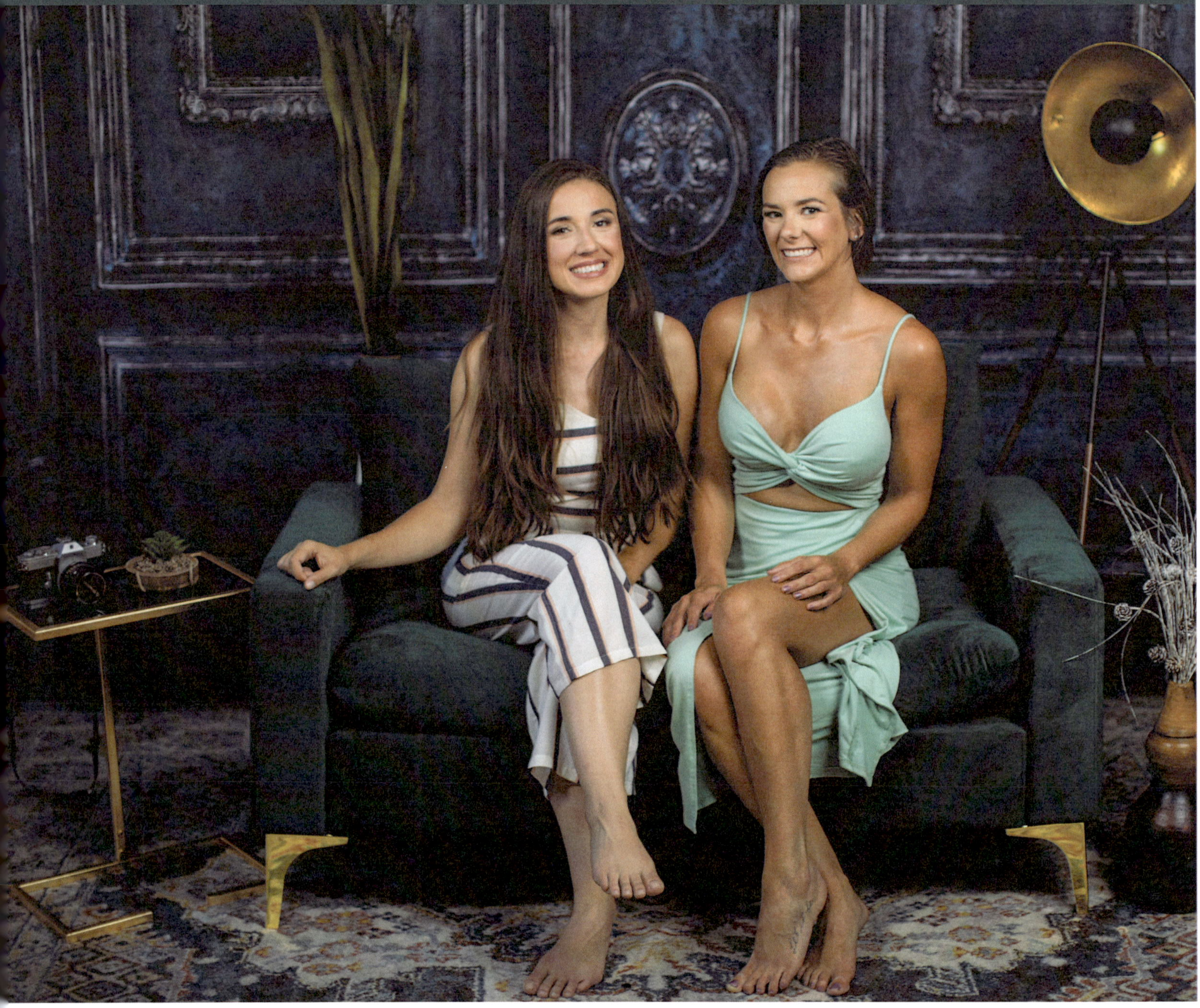

Founding Story

The Breast Cancer Confidence Project (BCCP) was founded in 2020 by Michaela Raes, who was diagnosed with breast cancer at just 28 years old.

Facing difficult treatment decisions and the physical changes that followed, she struggled with self-image—until a boudoir photoshoot with photographer Jolana Hollister helped her rediscover confidence in her body. Inspired by this experience, Michaela and Jolana launched the Breast Cancer Confidence Project to provide other women facing breast cancer with the same opportunity to reclaim their self-esteem.

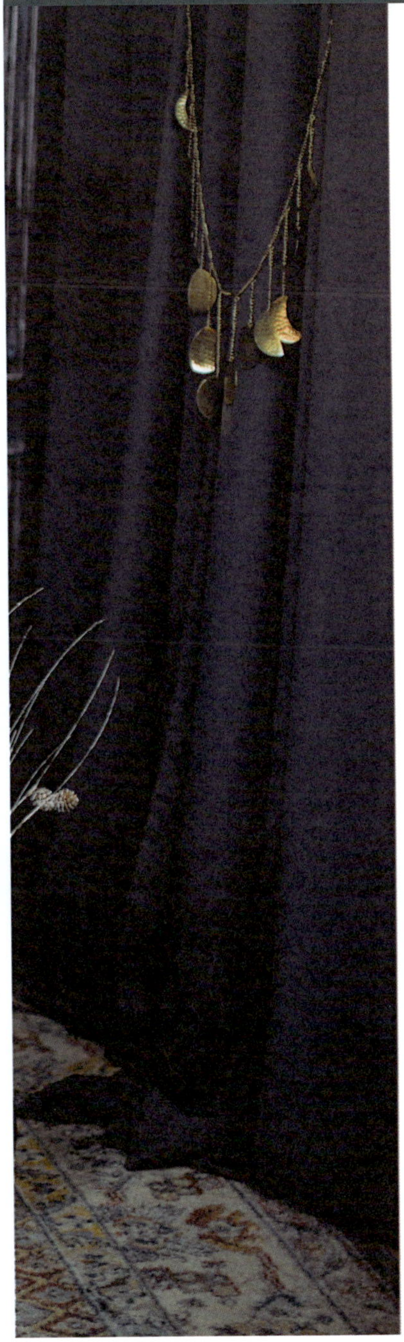

Since its founding, the organization has empowered survivors through intimate and supportive boudoir and portrait sessions, helping them redefine beauty, embrace resilience, and find confidence in their changing bodies.

With a growing community of Empowerment Ambassadors, the project continues to inspire women locally and beyond, ensuring that no one faces breast cancer without the support and encouragement to see themselves as strong, beautiful, and whole.

You Are Whole

You Are Whole began as a passion project led by Michaela and Jolana on behalf of the Breast Cancer Confidence Project.

Through their work with BCCP, they witnessed firsthand the profound impact that body image struggles have on breast cancer survivors.

They wanted to create something bigger—something that could reach beyond individual portrait sessions and remind survivors everywhere that they are whole, worthy, and beautiful.

That's when the idea of an empowering photobook was born.

Originally envisioned as a small, local project in Rochester, NY, You Are Whole quickly grew into something much larger.

A simple social media post seeking participants resonated far beyond their community, reaching breast cancer survivors and thrivers across the country—and across the oceans.

Moved by their words, Michaela and Jolana knew they couldn't limit this project to just one city.

They traveled across the U.S. to meet these remarkable women, capturing not only their portraits but the raw, unfiltered essence of their journeys.

Though You Are Whole has been two years in the making, its purpose extends far beyond the present.

This book is about healing wounds—some decades old—and rewriting the narrative around scars, survival, and self-image.

It is a testament to the power of women uplifting one another, a collaboration made possible by individuals across two continents who believed in this vision and contributed in the ways they could.

This project is proof that vulnerability can be a force for change.

That beauty is not defined by convention.

That through shared stories, we create space for healing, empowerment, and hope.

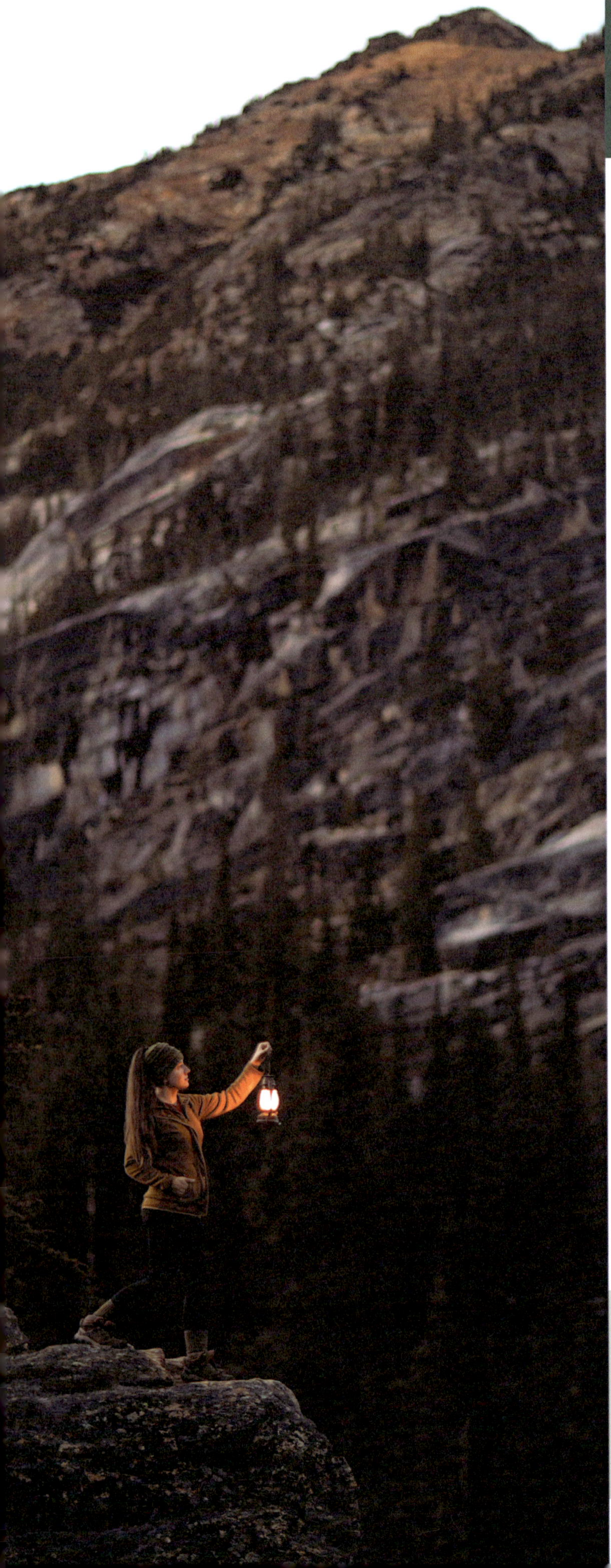

About the Photographer

Originally from the Czech Republic, Jolana has made Rochester, NY her second home.

She is a Rochester City School District & St. John Fisher University graduate.

After graduating college, Jolana pursued her love of psychology by working in the psychiatric emergency room, and her love of photography by starting her own business in 2014:
The Photography Experience, LLC.

Her work has been published both nationally and internationally in numerous magazines and exhibitions, and has received several awards.

With deep roots in psychology, Jolana finds photography to be therapeutic and healing in nature, and has built her business around it. Her mission in business is to provide experiences through artful photography that elicit a sense of belonging, empowerment, and connection to ourselves, others, and nature.

Outside of her business and Breast Cancer work, Jolana also volunteers her time to NILMDTS and other local non-profits, mentors women starting their own businesses, and shares her knowledge through teaching and speaking engagements throughout the community.

Her main goal in life is to eat, hike, and photograph her way around the world while fulfilling what she believes is our main purpose in life: creating genuine human connection while spreading beauty and positivity.

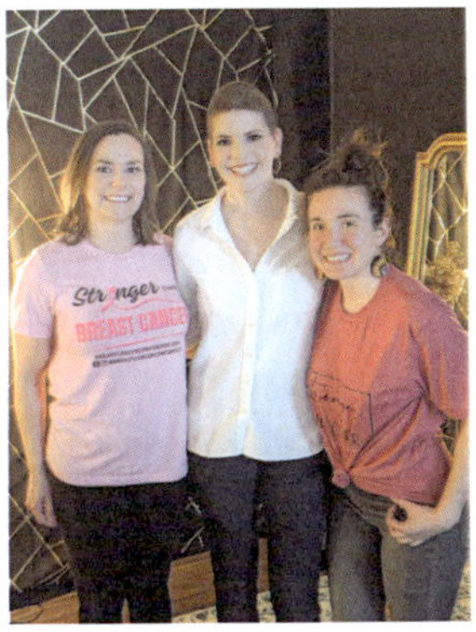
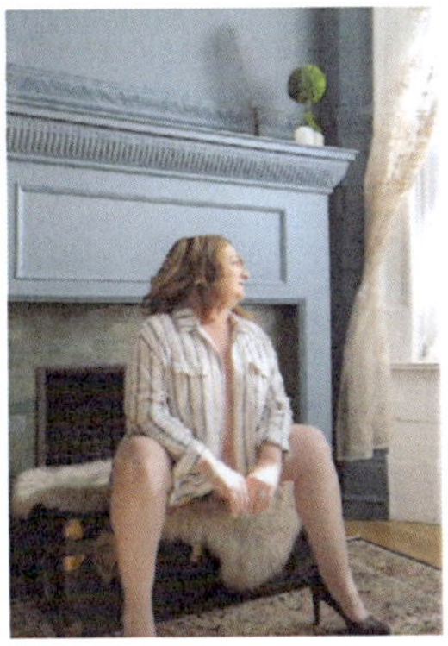
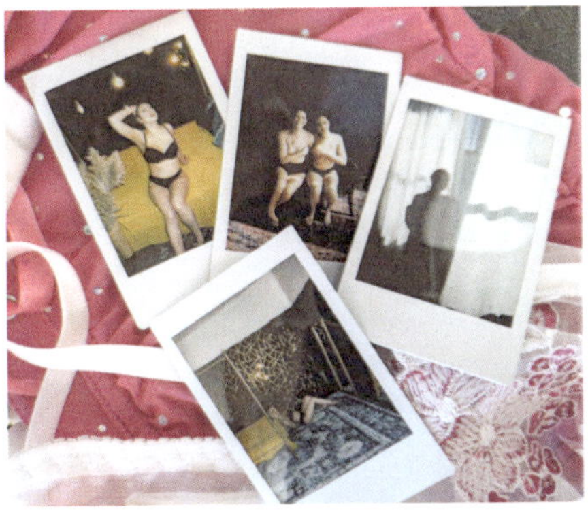
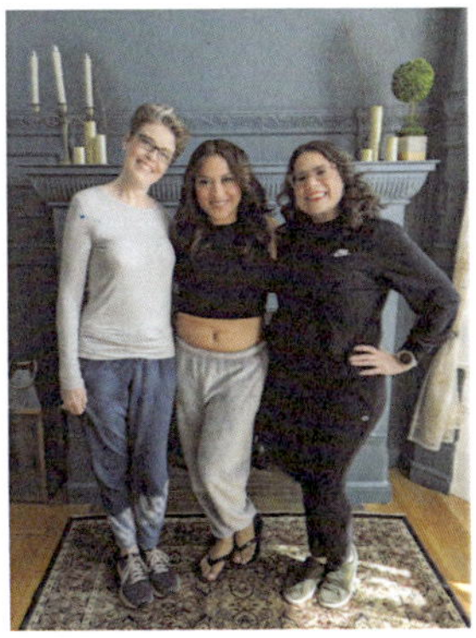
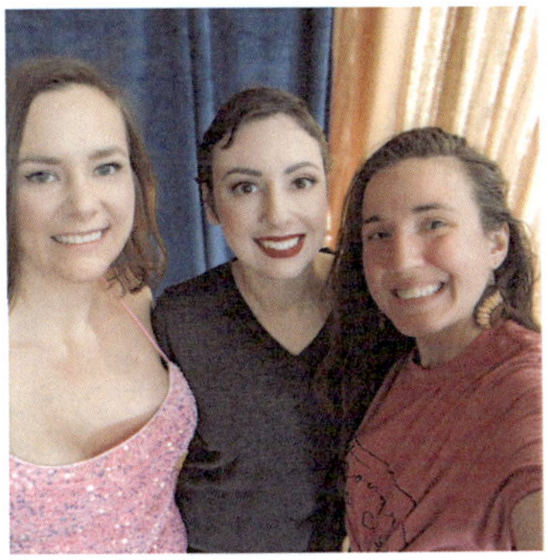
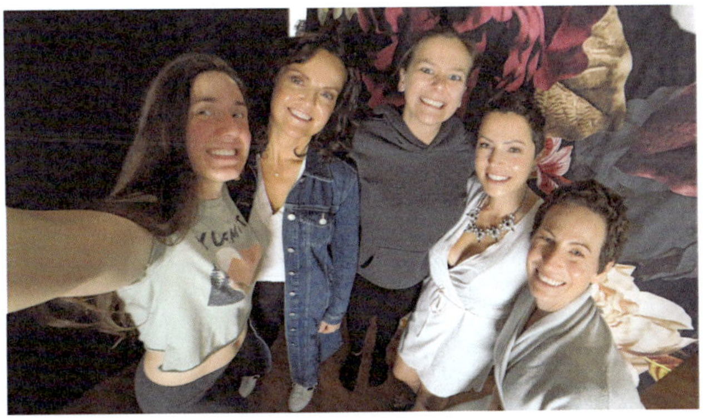
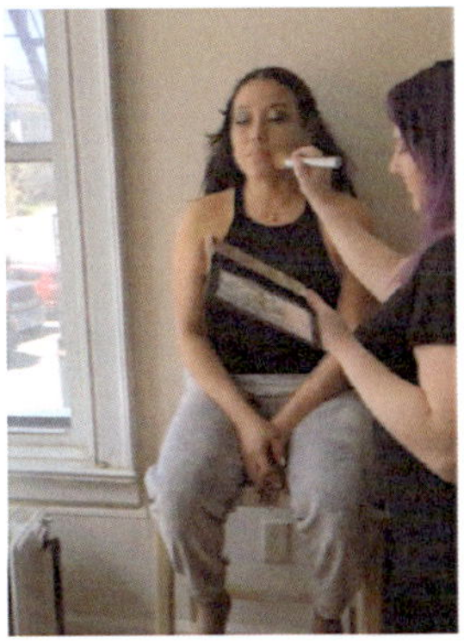

Behind the scenes

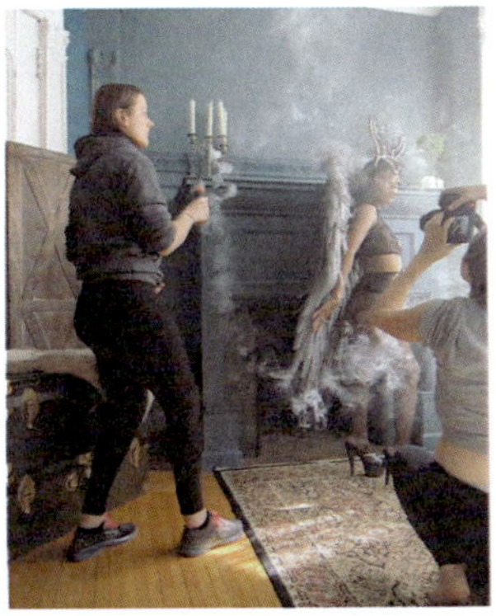
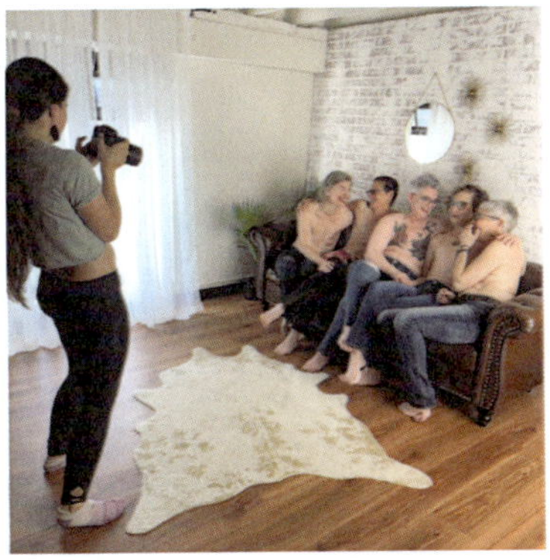
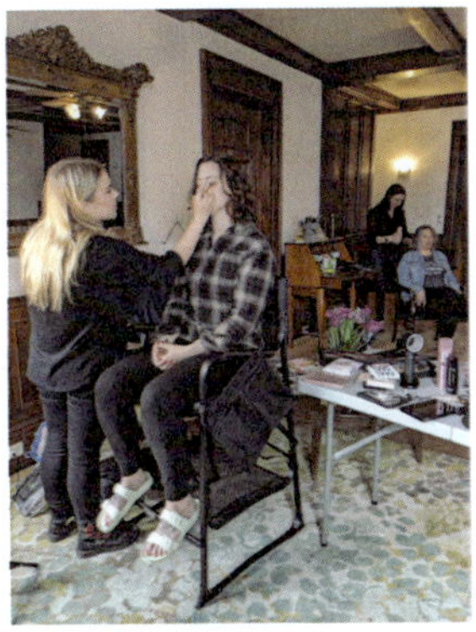
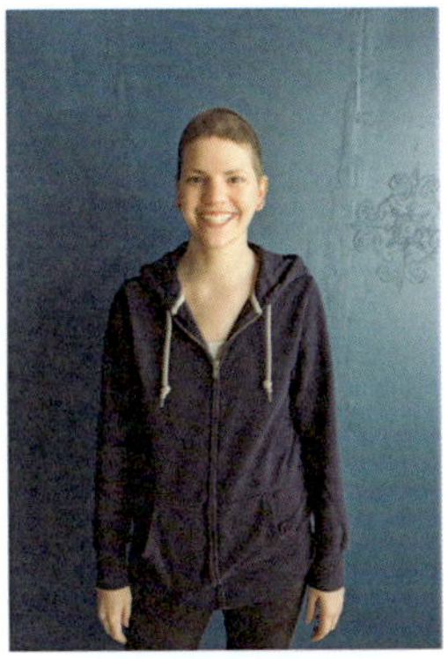
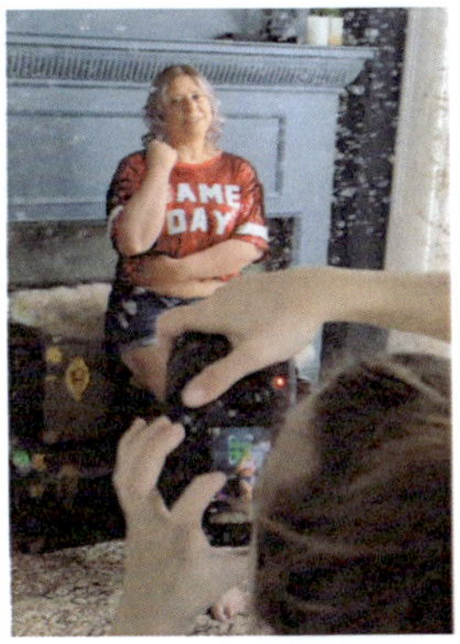
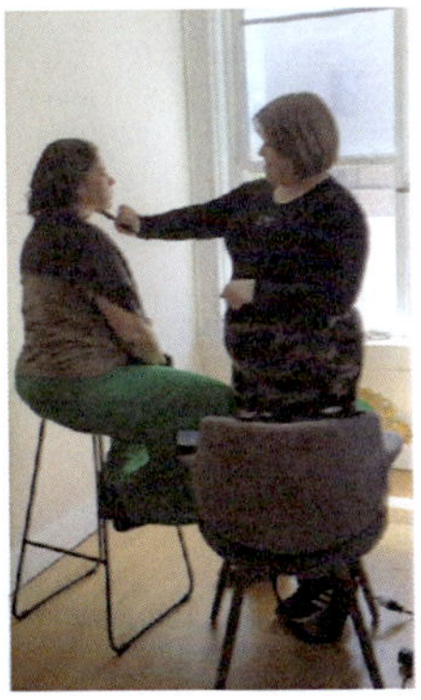
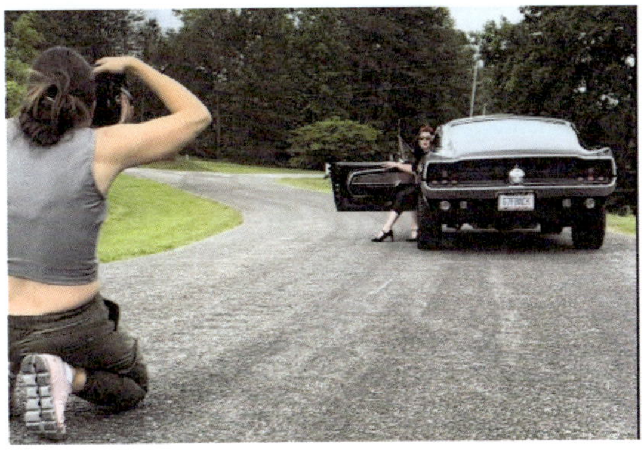
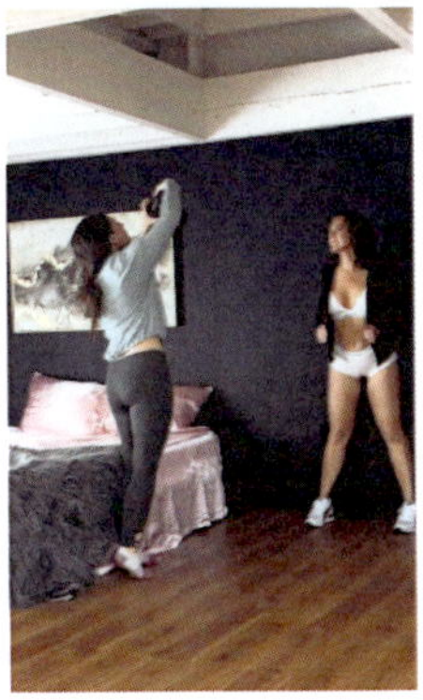
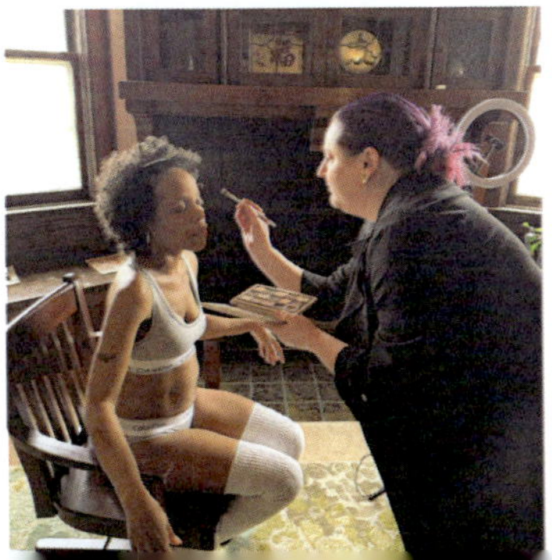
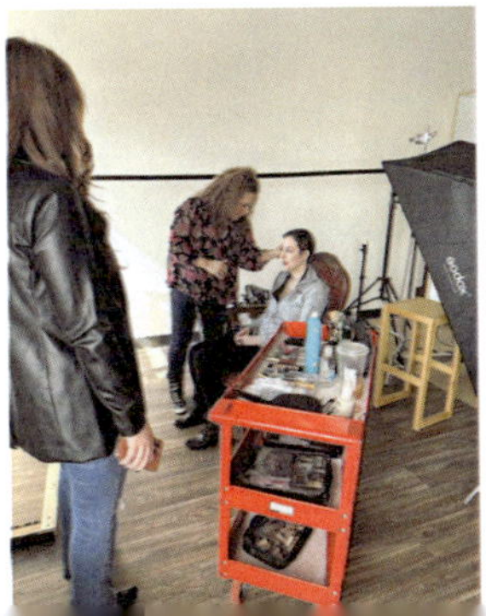
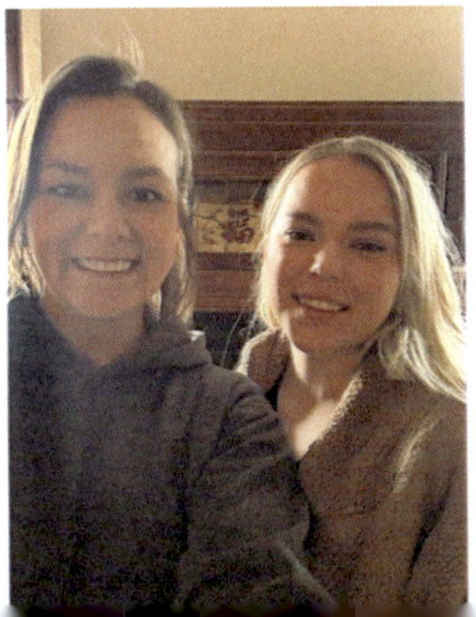
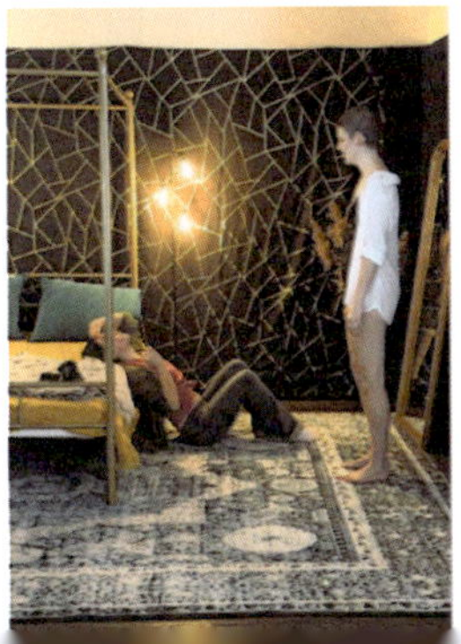

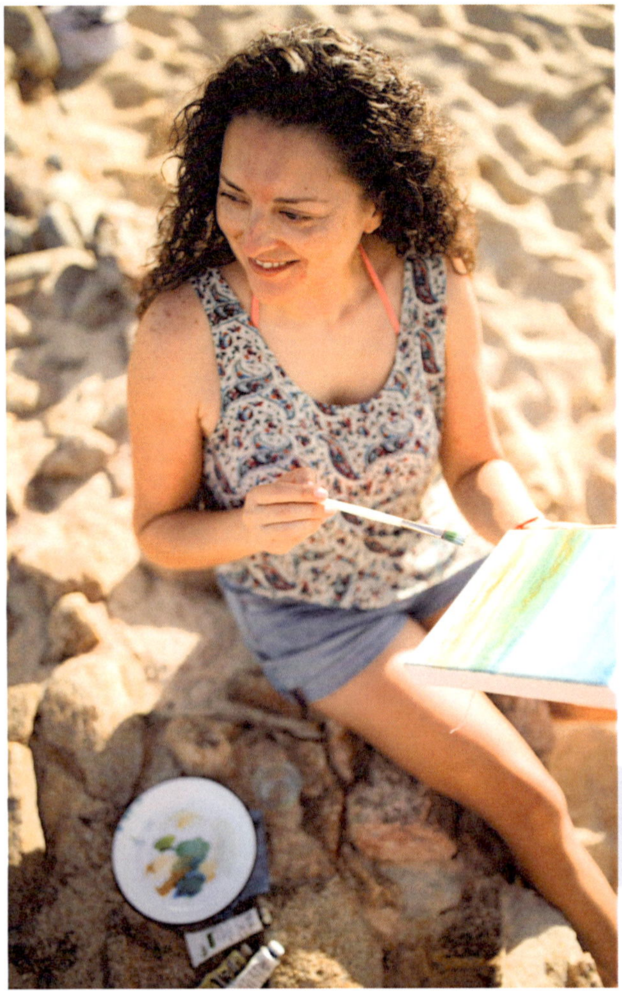

of a vast sky, whether illuminated by the radiant sun, the soft glow of a starry night, or the atmospheric weight of a somber setting. Her compositions are meticulously rendered on a variety of surfaces, each stroke and placement contributing to a cohesive whole that resonates deeply with the viewer's senses.

The power of Gibrana's artistic voice lies in its authenticity and lack of affectation.

Her expression is genuine and direct, devoid of pretense or the need to align with fleeting trends. It is an uninhibited flow of creativity that communicates with a compelling honesty, inviting viewers to connect with the inherent beauty she perceives and portrays in the world around her.

Her work stands as a testament to a pure and unadulterated artistic spirit.

About the Graphic Designer

Gibrana, a Mexican artist who resides in Los Cabos, Mexico,

channels her deep passion for art into a diverse range of mediums, including canvases that capture intricate details, delicate paper works, and expansive murals that command attention.

Her artistic sensibility transforms seemingly ordinary subjects – a solitary feather, the delicate flutter of birds, the intricate patterns of vegetation and seawaves, the expressiveness of faces and hands, the curves of human bodies, the grandeur of natural formations, and even everyday objects – into extraordinary visions of beauty.

These varied elements are harmoniously interwoven, frequently set against the backdrop

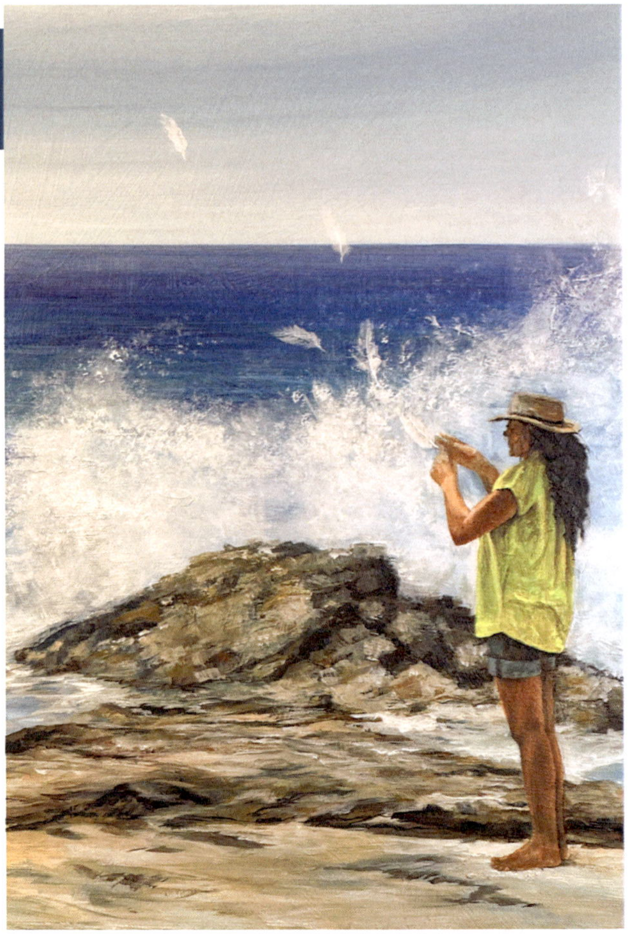

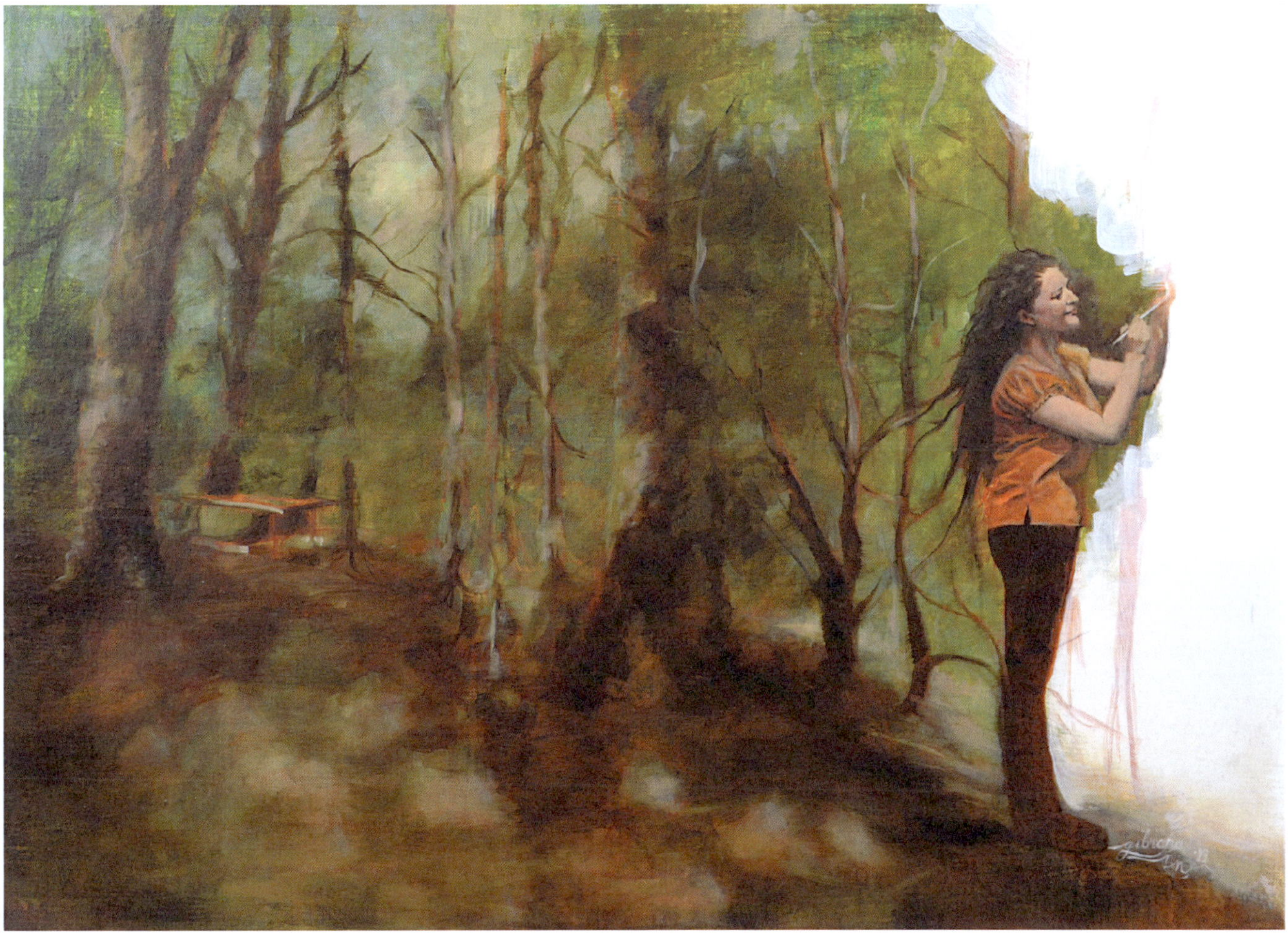

"La Historia de mi vida" (The story of my life)
2019
Oil on linen on wood
27.5 x 19.7 inches

This piece was created by Gibrana, whose own journey through ovarian cancer reminds us that we are all still writing our stories.

The blank space beyond the drawing is not empty; it is possibility. It is the unwritten chapters of your life, waiting to unfold.

For every woman in this book, and for every beautiful human reading it, breast cancer is just one part of the story.

There is so much still to be written. There is still so much to hope for.

To you holding this book right now:
Thank you for bearing witness.

May your own story continue with
courage, curiosity, and hope.

To Those Who Made This Possible:

You Are Whole was created in partnership with artists, makers, and space-holders who showed up with open hearts and open hands.

Whether through donated time or reduced rates, every contributor helped us create a space where survivors could feel seen, celebrated, and empowered.

To every hair and makeup artist who helped our participants feel radiant...

To each studio and venue that opened its doors...

You helped bring this vision to life, and your impact will be felt by every woman who sees herself in these pages.

Thank you for helping us reflect to every woman in this book that she is powerful, beautiful, **and whole.**

With Love and Gratitude,
The Breast Cancer Confidence Project Team

A Special Thank You To (By location):

CHICAGO

- *Hair & Makeup:*

Melanie's Makeup Artistry

- *Space:*

Feel Beautiful Photography

PORTLAND

- *Hair & Makeup:*

Jovana Combs Beauty

- *Space:*

Jamie Peterson Images

CHARLOTTE

- *Hair & Makeup:*

Adore Co Beauty

- *Space:*

Thank you to Katrina, one of our beautiful survivors, for sharing her home with us!

ROCHESTER

- *Hair & Makeup:*

Salon Crystallia
The ROC MUA
MJH Beauty
Leslie Whitney Hairstylist
Enhanced by Nature
BrittanyAnn Aesthetics
Kerrie Goodman Salon
Aesthetics By Andrea
Slay with MK

- *Space:*

The Photography Experience, LLC

PRAGUE, CZECH REPUBLIC

- *Hair & Makeup:*

Markéta Feigel